BLOW HIM

AWAY

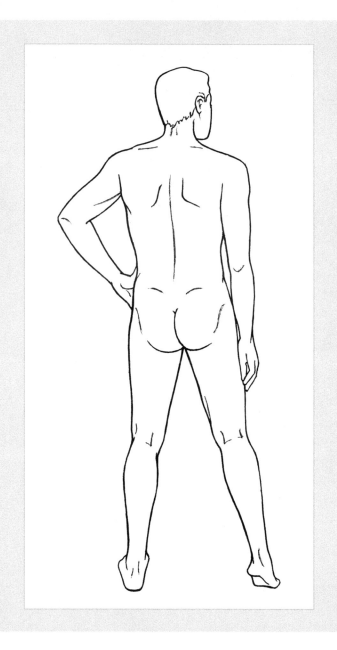

BLOW HIM

AWAY

HOW TO GIVE HIM
MIND-BLOWING ORAL SEX

MARCY MICHAELS

with Marie DeSalle

BROADWAY BOOKS NEW YORK

BROADWAY

DISCLAIMER: The instructions and advice in this book are in no way intended as a substitute for medical counseling. We advise the reader to consult with his/her doctor before beginning this or any other exercise regimen. The author and the publisher disclaim any liability or loss, personal or otherwise, resulting from the exercises in this book.

Broadway Books titles may be purchased for business or promotional use or for special sales. For information, please write to: Special Markets Department, Random House, Inc., 1745 Broadway, New York, NY 10019.

PRINTED IN THE UNITED STATES OF AMERICA

BROADWAY BOOKS and its logo, a letter B bisected on the diagonal, are trademarks of Random House, Inc.

Visit our website at www.broadwaybooks.com

First edition published 2005

Book design by JoAnne Metsch

Library of Congress Cataloging-in-Publication Data

Michaels, Marcy.
    Blow him away : how to give him mind-blowing oral sex / Marcy Michaels with Marie DeSalle.—1st ed.
       p. cm.
      1. Sex instruction for women. 2. Oral sex. I. DeSalle, Marie. II. Title.

HQ46.M52 2005
613.9'6—dc22

                                       2004051809

ISBN 0-7679-1656-5

20 19 18 17 16 15 14 13 12

Graze my lips, and if those hills be dry,
Stray lower, where the pleasant fountains lie.

—WILLIAM SHAKESPEARE,
"Venus and Adonis"

CONTENTS

On the Orgasm That Inspired This Book

A T SOME POINT, almost everyone asks me how I first made
the connection between speech therapy and oral sex. Did it just hit
me one day? Was it in a dream? Did one of my patients clue me into
the "side benefits" of my therapy? The answer requires a little back-
ground information.

My history and upbringing were far from sexually liberated. I
grew up thinking that a woman's place was in the home, and more
in the kitchen than the bedroom. To top that off, I married my first
boyfriend. If you had asked me where my G-spot was, I might have
pointed somewhere near my knee. "Naïve" doesn't begin to convey
how oblivious I was to the various parts of my body and their ability to generate sensual pleasure. The ever blossoming sexual revolu-
tion that swept across the nation barely touched me, incubated as I
was in a thankless marriage on the Upper East Side of Manhattan
with no career of my own, and not a single sex toy to my name. In-
explicably (I thought) unhappy, I finally went to see a psychiatrist.
As I sat in his nondescript office, he concluded that my problems
stemmed from a lack of sexual experience. I had been with only one

person, he reasoned, how could I know what I wanted? Taken aback by his prescription—"have sex with new partners as soon as possible"—I went out in search of a less wanton opinion.

Sexual liberation must have been going around that year, because psychiatrists numbers two, three, and four all gave me the same homework: take your sexuality into your own hands. Driven to the edge of despair by my unfulfilling marriage, I desperately, wildly, did just that—I took my sexuality into my own hands, and the rest of my life came with it. I divorced my husband, started my career as a speech pathologist, and got busy on the New York dating scene.

I was a woman on a mission. Having always been interested in helping others and in the power of speech, I decided to pursue an advanced degree in speech pathology. By day I went to my speech classes, and by night I broke loose on the grand ole isle of Manhattan. Professionally, I was studying with some of the most enlightened people in my field. Personally, I was dating some of the best lovers New York had to offer. I was thoroughly enjoying myself in both of these new worlds. The oral sex discovery resulted from an unlikely intersection of the two.

One day, on a trip to Atlantic City, I met a tall, pleasant fellow who took me around for the day. By that time, I was a little jaded. I had been dating for years by then, and thought I had seen everything. It was a fairly standard date—that is, until he gave me a good-night kiss that made my knees buckle and my stomach flip. My mouth, partially lost in his, moved into new realms, while my legs became heavy and sank toward the boardwalk. Sparks were sent flying all over my body, and an electrical current seemed to be running through my veins. Before long, we were inside my hotel room, and I was experiencing all-over body orgasms that challenged my definition of an orgasm as something with a beginning and an end. And he did it all night long without a gasp, a hesitation, or a slackening of energy.

Now this guy wasn't unusually charming or attractive. While his personality was fine and friendly, it was nothing to write home about, and his anatomy was entirely average. His tongue and mouth alone were responsible for my pleasure-fest, and immediately advanced him to the top of my list. So what transformed this mere mortal into an oral superman? Have you guessed yet? Of all things, Supermouth was trained as a *speech therapist*. I returned to my speech pathology classes in New York with a newfound enthusiasm.

This book is dedicated to sharing the secrets I learned in my years practicing speech therapy. They will help you gain a new mastery over your lips and tongue, enabling you to send shivers up your lover's spine. To make sure you get the most out of these techniques, I've included a handy, step-by-step guide to giving your lucky guy the best oral sex of his life.

So let's get you started.

BEFORE WE BEGIN: A NOTE ON SAFETY

The techniques set forth in this book are largely intended for the comparatively safe setting of a monogamous, long-term relationship. Of course they can be practiced on anyone, at any time, but they are meant to be experienced with someone you trust and know well. Though oral sex has been proven to be less likely to transmit HIV and other STDs than unprotected intercourse, the possibility still exists. Furthermore, if your partner has a bacterial STD, it is possible to contract it in your mouth or throat, or anywhere you have mucous membranes (including your nose). Keep in mind that the person performing these activities—doing the licking, sucking, or taking fluids into their mouth—is much more at risk than the person being licked, sucked, and generating the fluids. If you're getting intimate with someone you don't know very well, make sure you protect yourself with a condom or dental dam.

There are as many different kinds of protection available today as there are positions in the *Kama Sutra*, and some of them are designed to add the fun with flavoring and ribs. Before things get hot and heavy, find the products best suited to your needs that will allow you to be safe while exploring and expanding your sexual boundaries. Information on this topic abounds on the Internet (the Society for Human Sexuality at www.sexuality.org is a good starting place) and can also be found in numerous publications. Please do whatever is safest for you, so that you can delve into your sexual experiences with a truly carefree spirit.

BLOW
HIM
AWAY

Introduction

TO SUCK OR NOT TO SUCK: THAT IS THE QUESTION

MOST PEOPLE SUCK at performing oral sex, and for no good reason. This guide is based on the premise that oral sex can—and should—be outrageously fantastic *every time*. The poor quality of much oral sex being performed today can be baffling at first, but it becomes more understandable when one considers the factors involved. There are a plethora of psychological and social reasons that the tongue tickle hasn't been cultivated as a talent, but more often than not, a simple want of skill and knowledge is to blame.

When you engage in oral sex, you're taking the most delicate, vulnerable part of your lover's body—their genitals—and placing them between the most potentially vicious, animalistic part of yours—your teeth. The mouth is made to gnash, process food, and ward off harm. It's a wonderfully human quirk that we also use it to give pleasure.

Ironically, this distinctively human trait has been characterized by previous generations as dirty and uncivilized.

I don't need to argue here about the importance of great sex to the health of a romantic relationship. We've all seen TV shows and movies that portray sex and passion as über-racy, with bodies writhing in satin sheets under perfectly dimmed lighting, as if little elves had benevolently prepped the room for a perfect orgasm. But if sex and romance are overvalued, oral sex is all too frequently undervalued in the media and culture at large.

Still occasionally stigmatized as "dirtier" than straight-up coitus, the power of oral sex for sustaining and deepening a romantic relationship often gets overlooked. Sharing pleasure, as in intercourse, and *giving* pleasure have very different effects on a relationship, simply because they have very different effects on your partner. Being able to *give* pleasure to your partner, unselfishly and lovingly, can be more important, and plays a different role in your interpersonal dynamic. Oral sex is special in that it makes the other person feel cared for, tended to, and looked after. If actions speak louder than words, oral sex is like speaking through a megaphone when you tell your partner that you like and enjoy them.

Yet somehow, despite all this being so, most people don't perform oral sex as well as they could. But it doesn't have to stay this way—we can choose to raise the status quo. It just takes a little effort.

Oral sex must be performed properly to be effective and enjoyable. Unless your mouth is strong and controlled, there's a limit to how much pleasure you'll be capable of giving your lover.

Drawing on my experiences with patients, I can tell you that an average person trying to perform truly exquisite oral sex would have a very high likelihood of slackening their jaw control while they tried to keep up the muscular action of the tongue, leading the jaw to close in what could be a *very* painful mishap. The most pleasurable moves require a level of expertise that most of us simply don't have. When it comes to oral sex, we need more than a list of good ideas, no matter how tantalizing those might be.

Another problem with this "significant, beautiful" human act is that few people are willing to give oral sex its due. When it comes time to go down, some people flat-out avoid it, while others treat it like a chore. But in terms of sexual satisfaction, this is outright pleasure sabotage, given that many people view oral sex as actually *more* pleasurable than intercourse. It's time to face it, folks: *oral sex may be your most powerful sexual tool.*

Because your partner can lay back and focus all of their attention on the sensations you're giving him, oral sex is a highly memorable sex act. So, when things have been heating up and it's time to dive between the sheets (or unzip in the middle of the living room, as you prefer), before you perform oral sex, ask yourself how you want to be remembered. As someone who can give pleasure generously, or a skimp who's trying to hurry things along? To have your lover beating down your door for years to come, you need to give him more than one "oh-my-god, oh-my-god, oh-my-god" sensation—you need to be able to exploit the vast diversity of feelings that can be unlocked with just a tiny bit of muscular mastery, the oohs and aahs that are the bread and butter of great oral sex.

You may think you know everything you need to about oral sex, and that there's nothing a guide could tell you that you can't figure out for yourself. As for most guides out there, you're right. The majority of books about sex either recycle old material, or in their hunt for novelty come up with positions more suited for Gumby and Pokey than for you and your partner. But few of them prescribe the single ingredient that is widely needed: tongue and lip exercises.

Here you have the fruits of an entire field of study, developed by experts and researchers for many years, recontextualized and applied to oral sex for the first time. And it's only logical: out of all of the available specialists, wouldn't you want a doctor of the mouth to help you or your partner to perform oral sex?

In my practice as a speech pathologist, I've seen that what most people need is basic training. They need to strengthen and energize their mouths, lips, and throats so that they can perform *any and all* techniques with absolute comfort. Unless you're strong at your base, sophisticated techniques will never help you. In fact, students of sexual technique can (and have) hurt themselves or their partners while trying out new things. Giving your partner the best oral sex of their life isn't going to happen with just a couple of new techniques. You have to establish your muscular strength, refine your control, and *then* you can employ the moan-making, sheet-ripping, multiple-orgasm-generating techniques.

WHY SPEECH THERAPY IS OLYMPIC TRAINING FOR ORAL SEX

Thirty years ago, when I started practicing speech therapy, I would have laughed at the idea of me—or anyone else in my industry—writing an oral sex guide. Speech therapy belongs with dentists, orthodontists, and speech analysts, not Dr. Ruth, sex therapy, and dental dams . . . right? While it's perfectly true that most branches of speech therapy have nothing to do with oral sex, and while there may be a practitioner or two out there who's never even *had* oral sex, speech therapy nonetheless has designed techniques that will blow your partner's socks off (if they're still wearing them). So don't go swinging the gavel too soon. You can't judge a field of study by its unerotic exterior. The quality of oral sex increases so rapidly when these techniques are applied that they almost seem better for sex than they are for speech.

But you also can't chalk up these oral sex results to common speech therapy. Practiced at its most general, the entire field couldn't help you get a single sigh out of your lover. Except perhaps from boredom. Lots of speech therapy involves repeating monosyllables from a droning tape with a monitoring instructor. Great way to spend the afternoon, right? I didn't think so, either. In addition to being a speech pathologist, I was also trained as a myofunctional (literally, "muscle-function") therapist. Myofunctional therapy is the speech specialization that most directly applies to oral sex. In myofunctional therapy, muscles are gods: they can push and pull teeth around at their whim. They can bring a bone out of alignment, or they can bring one into alignment. It all depends on how the muscle has been trained to interact with other bodily systems. In the fight between muscle and bone (and these fights are taking place all over your body), muscles always win. They have an agency that no other part of the body can lay claim to. There's a reason people say they were "muscled" into doing something (although being "boned" has pretty straightforward connotations of its own).

You may think that your tongue is a soft, pink love muscle that simply rests in your mouth until you need it to chew or speak or get sexy. But it's the most powerful muscle in your body in terms of exerting force, and as any speech therapist can tell you, that little sucker is exerting force all day long. The tongue exerts a minimum of six (and a maximum of eight) pounds of pressure in your mouth *each* time you swallow. The average individual swallows one thousand times in a twenty-four-hour cycle. You don't need to be a math wiz to figure out that that's a *lot* of pressure—at least six thousand pounds a day—to be exerting anywhere in your body. And it's more than enough to alter the structure of your mouth and the placement of your teeth significantly.

There is a right way and a wrong way to place your tongue in your mouth. If we could feel just a little more of the six thousand pounds of pressure our tongues exert every day, most people would figure out how to place their tongues correctly as a matter of urgency. There's a part of the mouth that's designed to withstand the pressure of the tongue—the hard palate on the roof—but most people never use it. Instead, they rest their tongues between their teeth, in the bottom of their jaw, or even worse, against the backs of the top teeth. Over time, placing the tongue in each of these spots *weakens* the tongue and surrounding muscles. As you read this paragraph, where is your tongue in your mouth? If it's anywhere other than resting on the roof of your mouth behind (but not touching) the top row of teeth, your oral sex ability is being compromised. Try this experiment: read the rest of this book with the tip of your tongue *always* pressing against the hard palate on the roof of your mouth, without touching your teeth. Have it be the first thing you do each time you open this book. (For an illustration of where you should place it, turn to page 31.)

A poorly placed tongue impairs any and all uses of the tongue and mouth. Most people don't know that this is an issue—while performing oral sex, they might think that it's natural to feel strained, get lockjaw, or have a gag reflex. While kissing, they might think that it's equally normal to feel like they can't get their lips in the right spot. But all of these (and snoring!) are symptoms of a misplaced tongue.

Aside from these effects, the placement of these incremental bursts of pressure changes the shape of your jaw and the placement of your teeth, determines how free your tongue is to move in, out, and around your mouth, and influences how much energy it has. You probably didn't know that every time you swallow, you're either helping or hurting your greatest oral sex asset. You probably didn't even *want* to know that. But if you do want to give mind-blowing, satisfying, remembered-with-a-grin oral sex each and every time (and if you want to have fun doing it), you're gonna have to accept a few Tongue Realities.

Tongue Reality 1: Your tongue does not like it when you smoke. I know, I know, it's sexy (sort of) and it can be a way to bond with Mr. or Ms. Unapproachable Smoker, but the fact is that smoking isn't good for your tongue. A smoker's tongue tends to be lazy and lifeless, bulbous and placid. Your tongue needs to be an energetic, frontward, stand-up soldier, not a limp pile of mess-hall meat. Not to mention, smoking is very bad for you, so you wouldn't be getting rid of a productive pastime.

Tongue Reality 2: Your tongue needs exercise, too. You may think that your tongue gets a fine workout by eating and talking and frenching cuties, but usually quite the opposite is happening. Since most people don't even know the right position for their tongue, these activities actually weaken it by reinforcing bad habits. If you want a tongue that can lead wild excursions into intensely sensual experiences, you have to give it specific, controlled exercises. In chapter 4, you'll find some of the exercises to jump-start basic training for your tongue.

Tongue Reality 3: You don't know your tongue. Maybe you're lucky enough to have already gone to speech therapy (though you might not have recognized this as luck at the time). Or maybe you were even luckier and inherently assumed correct tongue positioning. But it's highly unlikely: out of more than 10,000 patients I've seen, not a single one walked into my office with their tongue correctly placed. Most of them didn't even know that there *was* a correct position for the tongue. But take heart—tongues are easy to get to know. They have simple needs that are easily satisfied. And you and your partner are going to get a lot out of this new acquaintance. Speaking of which, here's a list of side benefits to these exercises that could lure the biggest couch potatoes on the planet to open their mouths and exercise their love tools:

You'll Feel Better
Much of your body's tension goes into the face, neck, and shoulders, and stays there. We grind our teeth. We can't get our sinuses unclogged. We get short of breath sooner than we should, not from exertion but from not breathing properly. All these symptoms can be exercised away.

You'll Look Better
With your jaw muscles balanced, your tongue in the right place, and your swallowing patterns corrected, your face in repose will be at its most symmetrical and unstressed, so your features can appear to their best advantage. When you smile, talk, sing, or make love, you won't be contorted, look tense or appear worried, because your face will stop storing muscular tension—you'll be radiating charm instead of strain.

You'll Sound Better

Your voice will have a wonderful resonance, both richer and rounder than you've probably ever heard it. It will be sexier, more commanding. When you open your mouth to speak, your voice will have more tonal assurance, making people more likely to want to listen and respond to you.

Furthermore, if you snore (or if you're one of the thousands of unwitting youngsters who will begin snoring in the next twenty years), performing these exercises and keeping your tongue correctly positioned will eliminate the possibility of a single little snore—or even a midnight chortle—ever escaping your lips. When the tongue is positioned correctly, your mouth is physiologically incapable of snoring.

You'll Know More

You'll be able to check out a great deal about a prospective lover in advance—by the time you've completed the exercises in this book, a quick tongue reading, an assessment of face, mouth, and voice will tell you all that you need to know about a potential oral sex partner.

Now that you are familiar with these basic notions, it's time to start preparing you to deliver lifelong ecstasy. Many oral sex lovers are inadvertently lopsided—either they have lots of enthusiasm and lack the required skills, or they have some know-how but no panache. The following chapters are dedicated to making sure you're a well-rounded lover.

I

You Have to Walk Before
You Can (Unzip His) Fly:
Preparing Yourself to Find (and Swing)
Your Partner of Choice

If sex is such a natural phenomenon, how come
there are so many books on how to?

—BETTE MIDLER

IT WOULD BE a cause for celebration if we were born with the natural and intuitive set of sexual skills that we all pretend we have. Without stating it outright, our culture—via our parents, the media, and our peers—implies that sex and sexual skills should come naturally, with all but the most advanced techniques being instinctive. You'd never expect someone to hit a perfect tennis serve without lessons and practice, or to play a beautiful sonata on an instrument they've only touched a couple of times. Yet somehow, most of us come to maturity with the expectation that sexual skills will magically develop in the presence of our naked lover, that this lover will likewise experience a spontaneous onset of spectacular proficiency, and that it will all unfurl as smoothly as a movie montage.

Where do real-life Don Juans get their savoir faire? There's only one way: practice, practice, practice. Some people try to pick up tips from their friends, but while you may have an friend or two with information to spare, the likelihood is that you're dealing with what literary criticism calls an "unreliable narrator." (I personally stopped trusting the sexual knowledge of my peers when they asked me if my "cherry" had been "popped," but could not specify what this "cherry" was, nor exactly where it was located.) Truth: *real sex is awkward.*

The fact is, if you expect great sex to come naturally, you're in big trouble, and your partner is in even bigger trouble. Giving great oral sex is dependent upon being truly comfortable with the act, in good times and in bad. Real sex with live people is tricky—it smells, it squeaks, it gets stuck on some things and rams too quickly into others. People get injured physically (especially in the shower) and emotionally (especially in affairs), and on the whole, doing it probably causes about as many problems as pleasures. This doesn't mean that you should stop—in fact, most of us should be having more sex rather than less.* But it does indicate that we have a lot of false expectations surrounding sex, and these expectations take a lot of the fun out of sex without us even knowing it.

---

* A study conducted by the National Opinion Research Center, unlike previous (and subsequent) surveys, used a representative sample of the American population. They found that Americans have considerably less sex than is frequently portrayed by non-representative surveys (such as those conducted by condom companies), which are nonetheless reported as "news" in the daily media. The survey found that *one third* of adult Americans have sex a few times a year or not at all. This study was conducted from 1987 to 1994 with support from the government in response to scientific groups who could not find reliable information about American sexual practices. A comparably representative study has not been conducted since. ("Results of sex study by University researchers revealed in two books." *The University of Chicago Chronicle,* vol. 14, no. 4. Oct. 13, 1994.)

ACCEPTING THESE REALITIES WILL
MAKE YOU A BETTER LOVER

Sexual Skill Doesn't Come Naturally
Sure, the impulse to have sex is natural, and the heat of passion is sure to lend a little on-the-spot inspiration, but sexual skill must be learned and practiced like anything else.

Tell Him to Wash Behind His Balls
Genitals have a naturally pungent odor and taste. Some people love it, others don't. But you're in denial if you're surprised by it. If this is a concern for you, just take a bath or shower with your partner, instead of trying to skirt oral sex, or pretending to be comfortable going down when you're not. If you forge ahead anyway, your partner will sense your repressed discomfort, and the effort to conceal your true feelings will take the zest out of your performance.

A Funny Thing Happened on the Way to the Orgasm
Whether it's that funny slurping noise, a penis that veers to the right like it's catching a curveball, or a pubic hair in your eye, unexpected things are bound to happen during sex. Who can say what it will be? One woman I know started laughing while her guy was coming in her mouth, and it ended up dribbling out of her nose. Things like this are a natural part of an active sex life, so you might as well expect them and make sure to bring your sense of humor with you to the bedroom. Taking sex too seriously is a sure passion-killer.

Genitals Look Funny
Believe it or not, the overall quality of oral sex is still being compromised by people's shame and fear of genitalia. The people giving oral

sex are afraid to stare too much, because they don't want to make their partner feel uncomfortable, while their partner can barely even relax and enjoy themselves because they're so freaked out by someone sniffing around down there. Shocking as it is, this is occurring in the twenty-first century, and it's compromising the quality of oral sex. To overcome any vestiges of genital-fear, take a moment with your partner to really look at his genitals. Tell him why you want to do it, and make sure he feels comfortable with it first. Then look—really *look*— at all the different parts, and acknowledge that these are what you have to work with. An anatomically complete understanding of your partner's genitals will assure your subconscious that there is nothing "bad" or "dirty" or "scary" lurking in there anywhere.

"That was great. Really, it was . . ."

Most likely, no one's told you the truth about your sexual skills. It's a rare lover who openly communicates what they do or don't like, because they're trying to be nice. But withholding feedback is extremely counterproductive with regards to sex. The way people communicate about sex isn't even worthy of the term "miscommunication," because not only does withholding feedback send the wrong information (that you like something you don't, or dislike something you do), it actively obstructs future communication about sex. We're lucky consultants can't be called into the bedroom, because most people would be fired. The result? Very few men and women have been given enough feedback to develop a repertoire that works. And it's a damned shame. Since they haven't built up the strength and precision of their lips and tongue through a history of feedback and refinement, they develop a repertoire based on second-rate skills and subject every poor date they meet to it. As a loving pet owner thinks their cat or dog is absolutely unique among the breed, everyone—and I mean *everyone*—thinks they have great sexual skills. Meanwhile, most people report more than a few instances of less-than-satisfying sex every year. You do the math.

You don't have to pass out a comments and suggestions card afterward, but you do need to elicit your partner's feedback. A whispered "Do you like that?" during oral sex will produce more honest feedback than a "Was that good for you?" when the deed has already been done.

It's Not Just About the Orgasm

You don't have to make your partner come to have great oral sex. Great oral lovers are not orgasm-making machines, and if you treat oral sex this way you're not going to enjoy it—and neither will your partner. Aside from straining yourself, your orgasm fixation will actually distract you from your lover's subtle signs and signals. You don't have to frantically chase orgasms. The orgasm will come to you. Straining and stressing about how long it's taking your partner to come wards off a real orgasm like a snake scares a mare, so it's better to just let go of this expectation and enjoy yourself. Experiment and play—the light touch—will inevitably create more pleasure for your partner than strain or stress.

People who perform poorly at oral sex are usually hung up on one or all of these basic issues. But there's another related set of concerns that are a little more serious, and must be addressed for you to get the most out of giving—and receiving—oral sex. As much as oral sex is a matter of skill, it is also an issue rife with hang-ups and inhibitions for many people. These must be eradicated to unleash your greatest oral sex potential.

2

When Your Mind Spoils Your Head:
What Wrecks Oral Sex

NO MATTER HOW much you might try to convince yourself that you are a sexual cavalier and not a vulnerable human being, sex is an intimate act. It almost always brings up somebody's emotions. Oral sex, in some ways, is even more intimate. A Chinese proverb says, "If you save a person's life, they're yours forever." That's fine and well, but hair-pulling, moan-making, nail-sinking oral sex breeds its own strain of attachment, and it can be pretty fierce.

Partially because of the intense feelings of vulnerability, some people have a very hard time opening themselves up to receiving oral sex. At the thought of someone else fully exploring their genitals and witnessing their states of uncontrolled ecstasy, some people begin to drool, while others snap closed like a clam. (Personally, I drool.) Control issues (*After all, what might that other person do down there? Will they try to stick something weird in my [insert most feared orifice here] or do something else that I'm not prepared for?*), self-doubt (*Do I smell down there? What if I have to fart? What if I didn't wipe well the last time I . . . you know . . . ?*), and a negative body-image (*Are they noticing my love handles/cellulite/ass hairs/whatever aspect of my body I tend to de-spair over?*), as well as a plethora of other issues can take the fun out of oral sex faster than you can say the word "orgasm." And that's just on the receiving end!

On the giving end, performance anxiety and fear of being judged are chief among the pleasure-killers. *"What if they don't like what I'm doing?" "What if I get tired and need to stop before they've had an orgasm?" "What if I can't bring them to orgasm?"* And *"What if they're just pre-tending to like it?"* You may be surprised just how many people let thoughts like these crash their oral sex party.

While there is no magic potion to remove these inhibitions (other than drugs and alcohol, which are *not* long-term solutions!), there are some steps you can use before, during, and after your rendezvous that can help you to better relax and enjoy yourself. Being comfort-able and happy makes almost anything you do better, and this goes double for oral sex. In order to devote yourself fully to giving and receiving pleasure, you need to be as deep in the pleasure groove as you can get.

GETTING READY TO RUMBLE:
A DATING GUIDE FOR FABULOUS ORAL LOVE

For those of you who are perfectly comfortable with your body, have no trouble relaxing and getting down to business, and are 100 per-cent ready for action, skip this bit and go straight to chapter 3. For those of you who have been single for a while, tend to fumble with sexual tension, or simply feel that you could be better at relaxing and enjoying the ride, here's some information how to prepare your *en-tire* being for oral sex.

Before going out with a sexual (or soon-to-be) partner, most people spend time squinting in the mirror and picking out their most flattering clothes. Paying a little extra attention to your appearance and hygiene before a date is a natural inclination—and should be de rigueur if you're hoping for future dates—but the buck rarely stops here. All over the country, we go tearing through our closets looking for the "right" outfit, wrestling into one sweater just to run to the mirror and frown. "You're fat," the mirror says back to us, "and I'm not granting you any wishes." A new pimple or wrinkle just before a date has furrowed countless brows. "This big, ugly pimple next to my mouth looks *awful*—they'll probably think I have herpes! Maybe I should just cancel." These thoughts and feelings aren't restricted to ephemera—our more substantial physical "flaws" provoke even more nerve-racking thoughts. "My pubic hair is turning silver," an older friend confided in me, "and I don't know what's more painful: their facial expression when my underwear comes off, or plucking the damned things."

Fretting seems harmless, but how are you going to get comfortable and enjoy what your body can do if you've spent time before your date chastising it? The innocuous appearance of predate fretting is only skin-deep: it has very real consequences for sex and physical pleasure.

Shower Power

Being clean and sweet-smelling is a considerate gesture that says to your partner, "I want you to enjoy contact with my body," and it can boost your self-confidence. However, criticizing your body on *any* level will impede your oral sex performance, because how you feel about your own body will be played out in how you react to your lover's. It can also distract you from your partner's subtle signals and delay your own orgasms. Is being zitless and well-dressed worth that much? Is *anything*? Of course you should look nice for your date— but obsessive thoughts have a momentum of their own, and cannot be cast off as easily as clothing.

Consider limiting your preening time to around fifteen minutes— just enough time to cover the basics, not enough to nitpick. Use the rest of the time to prepare yourself psychologically to have fun and relax.

The Two Big Basics

These are very simple ideas, but disregarded by one and all. First, wear comfortable clothes. Not quite the jeans with holes and your favorite tattered sweater, but make it a rule to avoid tight or re-stricting clothes, and clothes that are out of character for you. If you don't look like yourself, you won't act like yourself. (Also, it's not a bad idea to leave the stilettos and fancy silks for a time when you may need the kinkiness.)

Second, use the time before your date to *relax* and *unwind*. If you're leaving work, take a walk around the block just to absorb the atmosphere of the neighborhood, or treat yourself to something that will loosen you up—maybe it's listening to music, getting a mani-cure, or going in a pet store and watching puppies tussle. Whatever it is, it needs to relax you. For more serious stress cases, it may take a ten-minute massage or a short yoga workout. No matter what your stress level is, though, there's one cure-all: breathing. The breathing exercises outlined in chapter 8 are among the best stress antidotes around. They cost nothing, take little time, and relax you utterly. But if you want to be giving off your most sexual vibes, there are some specific activities that will send sparks flying on contact, which will be discussed in chapter 10.

If you don't have time to relax and unwind before a date, simply pop into the bathroom and look at yourself in the mirror. Do you like yourself? If you don't get a resounding "Hell yeah, I'm awesome!" keep looking at yourself and just say out loud: "I like me." Say it until you start to mean it, and then you can go rock the world. Feeling good about yourself makes everything you do better.

THE RECEIVING END

This is supposed to be more fun than a roller coaster,
but I feel like I'm still waiting in line . . .

While the majority of this guide is devoted to *giving* oral sex, its raison d'être is to improve the quality of oral sex everywhere, for everyone. With this objective in mind, a little space is devoted here to people who expect to enjoy oral sex, but when the time comes, feel uncomfortable or disengaged. If you're already an oral sex hound, feel free to skip the rest of this chapter and move on to the next. But if you've had some disappointments in the area, stick around.

The Distraction Reaction
All you can think about is what you have to do tomorrow/some overdue project/an obligation, concern, or care of any kind.

This one comes first, because even if you have never experienced this problem, enough months of sharing a bed will bring it along. You don't have to have attention deficit disorder for your mind to wander to all kinds of unrelated subjects—and people—during sex. Receiving oral sex is a particularly likely arena for this because your participation is (usually) not required, and your mental attention even less so. Lots of people are disturbed by their wandering minds, because it seems to indicate a problem in the relationship. But this is usually not the case.

If you notice your thoughts repeatedly turning to the same obligation, concern, or care, take a deep breath first (always rule number one), and set a time to think about the issue. Not necessarily an exact time—no need to whip out your daily planner—but give yourself permission to completely forget about the issue until then. When the problem has been delegated to a future time slot, your present one will be free to delve more deeply into the twists and turns of sensual experience.

Another possibility is to spend more time unwinding before you get sexy—a hot bath, a little lounging around, a neck massage, or even taking a minute to appreciate your own innate sexiness is more than enough to break free of these thoughts.

All you can think about is an attractive person who is decidedly not *the one going down on you.*

Oral sex is particularly well suited to fantasizing. Because you can relax, and can't see much of your partner from most positions, it may well be Tom Cruise or Salma Hayek (or for the really imaginative, both) giving you the ride of your life.

Morally, other-person fantasizing is neither here nor there—but the fact that some people feel guilty about it is definitely here. If it bothers you, you may find that relaxing and focusing more deeply on your bodily sensations actually removes the *need* for fantasy of any kind.

One option is simply to realize that your mind is wandering, and to call it back to an awareness of your own body. Focus your attention on what you feel—this will make the oral sex better regardless. How do the sheets (or the carpet, or the dining room table) feel against your back? Notice your own body: How does the air feel on your skin? Are your nipples hard or soft? Rub your fingers lightly over your chest, noting the feel of your own skin. Sometimes we have to use simple measures to reintroduce ourselves to our bodies as a source of pleasure. Now refocus on the sensations your partner is giving you. Propping yourself up into a sitting position and wrapping your hands around the head of your lover can be a great way to let your body tell your mind exactly where you want it focused.

If you're still feeling distracted, don't be afraid to stop your partner and tell them that you're having trouble relaxing. If you make it *your* problem, most partners will be happy to help you relax. A little massage or foot rub can sometimes be more than enough, and may lead to some pretty exciting sex play on its own. You may get an invitation to talk over your thoughts, which is usually just the thing to send them away.

But if you decide to tell your partner to stop, be mindful—how you phrase it is very important here. You may be saying "this sucks" but for the time being it needs to sound like "I'm distracted." For now, take responsibility for your response. Later, frame your criticisms ("You need to . . ." "You aren't . . .") as suggestions ("I think I might like . . ." or "I want to try . . .") Remember: the person giving oral sex is just as vulnerable as the one receiving it.

All you can think about is what bad thing you might smell/taste like.

As hang-ups go, this one is the most needless, if only because it underestimates your partner's freedom of choice. You wouldn't blame yourself if your lover decided to use some slightly turned milk in their coffee or wanted to eat a plate of something you personally found distasteful. What your lover puts in their mouth is a conscious and considered decision. Granted, if you have herpes (or any other STD) and this is the cause of your concern, than you should *definitely* speak up. Otherwise, unless you're getting it on with a first timer, the likelihood is that your partner knows exactly what they're getting themselves into. And if they're going down on you, they clearly *want* to get into it.

In the event that this abstract "freedom of choice" talk doesn't do it for you, the other option is to simply tell your oral sex lover to "hold that thought" and go to the bathroom. If the courtesy of cleaning yourself will ease your mind, then it's well worth the interruption. Either way, if this is a concern of yours, make sure to do away with it before it does away with your good time.

All you can think about is the mound of cellulite/big pimple/strange and winding ass hair you discovered this morning after getting out of the shower.

Before a date, women and men alike will despair over one aspect or another of their physical appearance. And when clothes hit the floor, it's rare not to have a moment of exhilarating fear. Covering up our smells with deodorant, shaving off unsightly hair, clipping away our nails and repainting our faces with little brushes may make us more palatable to ourselves, but the message it conveys is that the natural body is unsavory and even gross. And how can you feel excited about showing your lover something that must be continually repressed? Something that has to be regularly washed and wiped because it is constantly getting itself gross again? And the licking is going to be happening where?

Aside from all the reasons, cultural and personal, that we may be self-conscious about our bodies, the important thing to remember is: we are *all* self-conscious about our bodies. Bottom line: the intense self-consciousness that comes with the first few sex events renders most people as blind as a bat. So you might as well enjoy yourself, and try focusing your energy on your partner and your pleasure.

When it's worth its sweat, sex temporarily lobotomizes our capacity for abstract, analytical, or critical thinking. And yet most people fear being criticized, analyzed, and examined precisely during these sensual and engrossing experiences. Sometimes I think my partners wouldn't be able to tell me how many fingers I'm holding up during sex (though the experiment has never seemed worth the interruption).

You're Afraid of What They Might Do

Remember that your partner has only one goal in mind: to give you pleasure. So let them succeed by really relaxing and enjoying yourself. If your partner is worth their salt, they will be trying to figure out your comfort zones by tentatively exploring areas and then waiting for cues from you to continue or not. Enjoy the preliminaries, and if you start to feel frozen up or like you're not responding, have them return to something you liked earlier. A little sigh or grunt will usually be more than enough to get your message across to a good partner. Others may have to be physically reminded of what felt good with a gentle nudge. The best partners will be on the lookout for shifts in your body posture, breathing, and muscle tension, and will change their techniques accordingly.

Another option is to nip your discomfort in the bud by showing your partner what you like. You can use your hands, mouths, and anything else you can think of to demonstrate. You can also use hot, sexy language to describe it in a way that will build anticipation.

You should never have to feel concerned or tense about what your partner might do to you during oral sex. A few words, and sometimes just a subtle movement, are enough to give them the indications they need for what makes you comfortable and what you like.

Now that you're truly prepared, inside and out, to give and receive oral sex (and perhaps do both simultaneously), let's suit you up with the skills you're going to need to capitalize on this potential for a deeply satisfying sensual exchange.

3

Initial Tonguework for
Lingual Love

PREPARING YOUR MOUTH AND TONGUE
TO MEET YOUR PARTNER OF CHOICE

THE BEST PREPARATION for any mouth about to engage in oral sex is a good, thorough toothbrushing that addresses every side of the teeth (outside and inside, from the ridge to the gum line) with equal enthusiasm and plentiful toothpaste and water. Move the toothbrush over your tongue, use a mouthwash, and when it's all over, run the toothbrush over your lips to remove any dry, chapped skin. A soft, clean mouth is a much more welcome pleasure-giver. If you're with a new partner and not using a condom (though I suggest you do), keep in mind that the lip-brushing can create minute cuts, on and around the mouth and raise your susceptibility to STDs.

Before beginning the exercises in the book, take a moment to isolate and define the problems you might be addressing.

1. *Lockjaw.* Your jaw is gripped by tension, set in one position, so your tongue is allowed no free play. (This can be a particular problem for lispers.)

2. *The Tooth Monster.* Lack of jaw control can mean that your teeth get in the way, snagging on things that they shouldn't and making what should be a tender, erotic moment seem like an operation without anesthetic.

3. *The Drowning Pool.* You produce too much saliva, which gets in the way of your breathing properly and keeping up a steady, even, controlled stroke.

4. *The Tongue Depressive.* Your tongue is sluggish, lazy. You can't flick it lightly, catching those sensitive spots at the right time and with the right pressure.

5. *Flabby Tongue.* Your tongue is bulbous, large and flaccid, with no flexibility and no tonal quality. For all the good it does your partner, it might as well have rolled itself up into a ball and curled itself away to hibernate for the winter.

6. *The Big Gag.* You don't know exactly why, but you're gagging. And you thought only collard greens could do this to you! But don't worry, it can be easily fixed without years of psychotherapy.

Everyone has a different relationship to oral sex, and while many of these problems may have psychological and cultural components, developing your skills and sense of confidence toward oral sex will help give you an overall sense of well-being. If some or all of these items are issues for you, you might want to jump ahead to chapter 6 and take the Oral Sex Fitness Test. Then, when you have a sense of how fit your tongue is in general, you will know how often to perform the exercises needed to strengthen the following areas and eliminate these problems for good.

The techniques you're working to attain will create a firm foundation from which you can build more advanced skills. They won't automatically make you a great oral lover, but they will give you all the tools you need.

Jaw Control. So you can open your mouth as wide as necessary, without straining.

Proper Breathing. Learning how to breathe in and out of your nose, so you don't run out of breath while your mouth is busy. You'll eliminate one more distraction, and make it that much easier to concentrate on the magic that's passing between you and your lover.

Easing the Tension. Oral sex involves more than just your mouth. Learning how to relax your neck and shoulders, your knees, your fingers, your whole body, will contribute greatly to your being able to focus all your enthusiasm on the matter at hand.

Swallowing. Using your whole throat to swallow releases the constrictions in everything that's above it—tongue, sinuses, nasal passages.

Tonguemanship. This is probably the most sensitive, sensuous part of your body. But you have to know how to use it—and you have to get it into shape.

GETTING TO KNOW YOUR TERRIFIC TONGUE

The next time you're in the bathroom, take a look at your tongue. Most of us think of our tongues as one unit, but the tongue has four distinct sections that you will need to familiarize yourself with in order to move your tongue techniques into second gear. These are: the tip (the position of the tongue nearest the teeth), the blade (the point just below the alveolar ridge), the middle (the section that touches the roof of your mouth beyond the alveolar ridge when you arch your tongue), and the back (the part that falls away from the roof of your mouth in an arched position).

Your tongue is the largest and most powerful muscle in the body, and distinguished from other muscles by its ability to flatten and point itself so dexterously. By its capacity to flatten and lengthen, or sharpen and point its tip, as well as its ability to alternate between heavy and light exertions of pressure, the tongue is custom-crafted to administer oral sex. There is nothing in your local sex shop that can do all this. To boot, the tongue has a smooth underside, as well as a rough top texture "for their pleasure."

The Spot
The first step in developing your tongue's strength and precision (directly connected to its ability to give pleasure) is to identify the Spot. This is a particular place on the roof of your mouth where you will need to place your tongue for the majority of the tongue- and lip-strengthening exercises in this book. To find it, insert your (clean) finger into your mouth so that you're touching the place where the backs of your top teeth meet the gums. Trace your finger from here to the spot where the roof suddenly drops to another level. This slope is known as the *alveolar ridge*.

Remove your finger and start playing with your tongue. See how sharply you can point the tip. It needs to be more like a pencil than an eel. The sharper you can make the tip, the more delicately and precisely you are going to be able to stimulate your lover. When you have made your best possible point and identified the tip of your tongue, place the tip *only* on the drop-off (or alveolar ridge). Don't let your tongue touch your front row of teeth, and make sure that it doesn't fall beyond the ridge.

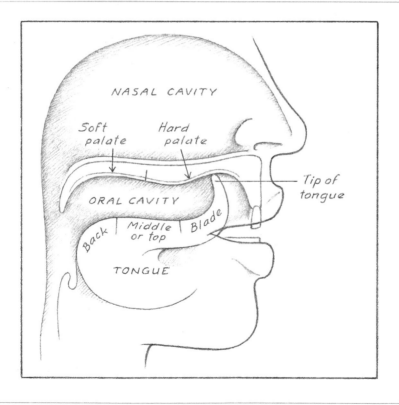

The Spot: Perfect Placement for the Tongue

Keeping your tongue in this position will stop it from changing the position of the lips, something the tongue is notorious (in my field anyway) for doing. Think of your tongue as a hammy actor— it's always trying to get past, distract, or upstage your lips and jaw from their function. But worse than that, it can also take energy away from the lips. So put that tongue in its place.

Aside from enabling you to participate in the exercises, placing your tongue here can stimulate the blood supply to the brain, increasing concentration and mental clarity. To do this, keep the tip of the tongue pressing up into the Spot, and let the middle of your tongue come up onto the roof of your mouth *without* changing the tip's pressure. Only the middle should be pressing into the curved top of the mouth. The back of your tongue should still be hanging down into the back of the mouth. Holding this position will help you become more composed and clear-minded. It requires a little practice to keep your tongue here (about as long as teaching a dog to "stay"), but this position gives back ten times what you put into it.

4

Kissing

PERHAPS BECAUSE KISSING on TV and in movies is immediately passionate, kissers tend to try to copy what they've seen. But the art of kissing cannot be reduced to pucker-and-lunge. There are as many different kinds of kisses as there are people kissing, each with its own particular combination of pressure and pace.

The ancient Indian *Kama Sutra* was aware of this, devoting an entire chapter to kissing and identifying fourteen types of kisses. In our culture today, we seem to have forgotten just how varied kissing can be. We know about the peck, the lip kiss, and frenching, but all the in-between is frequently overlooked, and kissing itself is frequently rushed through as a trifling preliminary.

Partially, this may be because most of us don't know how to use our mouths and lips in ways that produce a variety of erotic, pleasurable sensations (although erotic desperation definitely takes some of the blame). Whatever the cause, maximizing the pleasure afforded by your oral kisses will enhance all your lingual caresses, and alert your partner to the pleasures in store for them.

The most common complaints I hear concern half-lipped, lifeless kisses, so we'll address these first. Complaints about this kind of kiss range from disengagement ("I felt like she was just poking and pressing her lips around mine") to actual confusion ("It seemed like he was trying to whisper something really close to my mouth, like right into it. . . . Then I realized he was *kissing* me.") A very common phenomenon, this kind of weak kissing results from the individual's using only a small portion of the outer lip to kiss, instead of their full lips (including the smooth insides of the lip). The result is a dry kiss that feels more like lip bumper cars than an expression of passionate tenderness. The exercises in this chapter can help you use your full lips to create a maximum sensation of pleasure when you kiss.

COMING TO GRIPS WITH YOUR LAZY LIPS

Though they take over completely during kissing, lips are a primary point of contact with your lover during all of oral sex, so they must be as exquisitely soft and pleasing to the touch as possible. These kissing exercises must be as devoted to developing a velvet touch as they are to extending and strengthening lip movement. While developing mastery over the movement of the lips is extremely important to help them create a wide variety of sensations on cue, you do not want to tone your lips so much that they become firm or traditionally muscular.

To keep your lips soft and inviting, make sure that you *never* perform lip exercises with tense lips. Pucker and tap your lips gently with your index finger. How soft do your lips feel? This is how they should feel when you perform the lip exercises. Avoid tensing your lips when you go through the motions of each exercise. For the first week of practice, you should do all of the exercises in this book standing in front of a mirror, so that you can be sure that the correct part of the lips and mouth—and nothing else—is moving. In the beginning, you should do each exercise separately, with a five- to ten-minute break in the interim. After the first week, the exercises can flow into one another. Each exercise should be performed every day for seven days; then you can switch to every other day for an additional week to train the muscles to remember their new skills.

Kissing Exercises

Pucker Up

With your tongue on the Spot (see chapter 3), push your lips all the way forward until they open and roll their insides out, sticking as much of the inside of your lips out as possible. Then, keeping them fully extended, open and close your lips, bringing just the fleshy parts together to form a small circle. Touch them together five times. Practicing Pucker Up may make you look a little silly, and a lot like a fish, but trust this exercise—it will put you far ahead of the game by helping you find the correct positioning of the tongue and jaw.

This exercise acquaints you with the soft insides of your lips. When you perform it, notice what potential the lips have to create soft, delightful sensations (lip implants are popular because they promise exactly this sensation). But in order to deliver it, make sure to note the difference in texture between the soft, glossy inside and the drier outside of the lips. Many people make the mistake of firming up the lips, and kissing with only their rough outside edges. This misses out on the moist inner lip's inherent kissability. (You can feel how unstimulating this is if you simply close your lips and slightly roll them in between your teeth so that only the outer lip is exposed.) This part of the lip has no friction or engagement, both of which are absolute necessities for an erotically stimulating kiss.

However, others make the mistake of rolling the lips out too far. This results in the "I felt like he was eating my face" sensation. When you kiss, the other person should be able to feel *both* the rough and glossy parts of your lips, and never just one or the other. Similarly, during oral sex, the entire lip should be used for greatest effect.

Another issue that significantly impacts kissing and oral sex is the *strength* of the lips. Most of us never consider the lips as muscles, but lip strength is an extremely important factor for any kind of lingual caress. Pucker Up identifies and prepares you to use your entire lips, but if the muscles are weak the effect won't contribute much to your kiss. In order to give a really memorable, arousing smooch, your lips need to be strong and under your control. One exercise for this is called E like "Eat," O like "Swoon" (you can use your imagination for what kind of "eating" this refers to).

E like "Eat," O like "Swoon"
With your tongue on the Spot and your teeth together, look at yourself in the mirror and pull your lips as wide apart as they can possibly go. Place the pads of your index and middle fingers against the teeth, and start saying "eeeeeeeeee." Not "ehhhhhh," like "elephant," but a strong, sharp "e" like "eat." Keep looking in the mirror to make sure that your lips are the only things moving (i.e., don't move your jaw, neck, or tongue) and that they are stretched widely enough so that they aren't touching your fingers. Hold your lips in this position for a count of ten. When you're ready, remove your fin-

gers and pull your lips into a tight little circle with the insides of the lips pressing forward—as if you were trying to touch someone else with the smooth insides of the lips—and say "oooooo" like "swoon." This will strengthen your lips, as well as the surrounding muscles.

These two exercises are important to perform for ten repetitions every day for a week, because the more advanced exercises later in the book will build on them.

Once you've mastered the exercises specifically for kissing, you can start practicing those intended for the much more powerful king of kisses: oral sex.

Advanced Lip Exercises for Kissing

The Saltwater Pump—Front

Pumping exercises increase your lip dexterity. Put one teaspoon of salt in half a glass of warm (not hot) water. Pump a mouthful of this back and forth behind your upper lip. Allow the shape of your lip to be changed by the pressure of the water moving in and out. Perform this for a full minute, pushing the water as far as it will go without opening your lips. The presence of the salt will make you aware of the exact places your lip expands with this exercise. Take note of just how much your lip can actually stretch, because you'll be using the insides of your lips extensively in kissing and manipulating the finer points of your lover's anatomy. You should be using a half a glass of water to complete this exercise through a series of three to seven mouthfuls (depending on the size of your mouth). Do this three times a day.

Remember not to swallow the water. Stand nearby a sink or receptacle so that you can spit it out.

The Lip Massage

Whereas the Saltwater Pump softens the deeper tissues of your lips, performing the same motions with air softens the very surface of the lips, especially the delicate boundaries where your two lips touch. It will also help you gain control over this crucial area for oral sex.

Using your breath instead of water, push air behind your upper lip as firmly as you can. Again, do not tense or engage the lip muscles, but allow them to be moved and stretched by the power of your breath. Do this repeatedly ten or twelve times during the day.

The Saltwater Pump—Side

Using the same ratio of salt to warm water as in the Front Pump, push the water outward against the cheeks. Allow your cheek muscles to relax completely, then slowly push the water completely into them and maintain the position for a few seconds. Let the water fill back into the mouth gently, with still further relaxation of the cheek muscles. Alternate forcing the water in and out of the cheeks in this manner. Do this five times a day, filling and emptying twice each time.

Monkey Face

Slowly force salt water behind the upper lip, gradually building up pressure until the lip is completely rounded out. Make sure that the lip muscles are completely relaxed. Do this five times in a row, then perform the same process on the lower lip.

Try this again using air to reach the subtler musculature. The reason for doing both is that while using water makes the lips more flexible, air makes them tangibly softer. Taking some air into your mouth, force it gently into your upper lip, as if you are blowing up a balloon. Hold to the count of ten, five times in a row on the upper lip, then the bottom lip, and then both.

The Jug of Plenty

This exercise will give you some of the most memorable lips on the planet. To perform it, you need an empty plastic half-gallon jug (or container of equal size and weight) and about four or five feet of string. Good cotton string is highly preferable here to dental floss or thread.

Place the jug on the floor, and tie the cotton string through the handle so that you can lift the jug off the floor with the string. Put one end of the string in your mouth, and bend over so that you are looking directly down at the jug. Lift the jug off the floor by puckering your lips and using them to pull the string into your mouth. Do not bite the string or use your teeth. (And you may want to close the blinds!)

Some people start to suck straight in, as if they were pulling in a long piece of spaghetti. Instead, actively use the *inner* part of the lips to pull in the string, hold it to the roof of your mouth with your tongue, and then use your lips to pull in the next segment. You don't need to continue lifting until the point of standing up—six or eight inches will do. Your face should remain parallel to the floor. Lift and lower the jug ten times (each time should take only a few seconds).

Be very careful when taking the string into your mouth. Do not perform this exercise haphazardly or while rushing.

Button Up!

The purpose of this exercise is to get the muscles of your lips to strengthen by working against themselves. The lip muscles are toned when they are forced to adapt to increased stress.

For this exercise, you will need a button between the size of a dime and a quarter and a piece of string as long as your arm. Thread the string through the button, and tie the ends of the string together.

Pull the button with one hand and a place on the string with the other until the doubled string is stretched taut. Place the button in your mouth, and position it equally between the top and bottom lip (but not touching your teeth). Holding the button with your dominant hand (left for left-handed, etc.), hold the string so that it is perfectly straight and even. Begin to pull your hand slowly away from your motionless head with steadily increasing force.

The button will attempt to escape your mouth by opening your lips—don't let it. Pull harder until you find the point where you lose the button. Try to remember how far away your hand is when it pops free, so that you can set your goal for the next time just beyond that point. Do this five times a day for seven days, then three times a day for another seven.

These exercises all help to make the lips supple and soft, while maximizing their tone and energy so that they never tire of giving your partner pleasure. The energy you put into your lips here will show up in tenfold when it's time to give some luscious licks and kisses.

Tongue-Tied

Let's refine your control and fine manipulation of the tongue. For french kissing, an excellent exercise is to look in the mirror and to bring your tongue fully to a point. Would *you* want to kiss your tongue? It should be a healthy pink. If your tongue looks whitish, or even yellowish, make sure to use a tongue scraper after each brushing.

Stick out your tongue and bring it to a point without touching the teeth or lips. Hold it in this position and make a mental note of its size and shape. Now relax and widen the tongue as much as possible, still without touching the teeth or lips. The first time you perform this exercise in the mirror, you may be surprised by just how versatile your tongue really is—it can stretch from a point less than half an inch long to four times that size without touching the teeth or lips. The concept of your tongue as a free agent, moving independently of your teeth and lips, is particularly important for oral love—even crucial. While kissing, allow the tongue to move independently, but avoid making it sharp or pointed (at least until kissing has become extremely passionate and aggressive). Remember that a soft, wide tongue is much more inviting than a darting poker, and that each minute change of your tongue shape will be felt intimately by your partner.

ORAL ETIQUETTE

> Straight men need to be emasculated. I'm
> sorry. They all need to be slapped around.
> Women have been kept down for too
> long. Every straight guy should have a
> man's tongue in his mouth at least once.
> —MADONNA

Allow me to say it for you: *What?* How could someone as sexually open and liberated (at least ostensibly) as the superstar Madonna have such bitter, resentful feelings about men and kissing? But more important: why should there be any relationship between kissing and being "kept down"? The statement is clearly emotional, relating the way having a man's tongue in her mouth made Madonna feel. It seems highly likely that somewhere along the line a tongue went too far and too fast, and what should have been a pleasurable experience became distasteful, unpleasant, and perhaps even disrespectful.

Though Madonna's feelings as expressed here are extreme, I would venture to say that the feeling of a tongue playing tonsil hockey in your throat is not an altogether uncommon experience. Madonna may see it as a patriarchal show of dominance, but the likelihood is that her kissing partner(s) was just unskilled and too nervous (after all, he was kissing Madonna) to control the speed, force, and extension of his tongue. Furthermore, this plunging kissing style is not limited to the male sex.

This style of kissing is the tragic downfall of the overzealous kisser. Inadvertently making someone suck on your tongue is definitely one way to put the flame of passion right out. It does not necessarily increase your partner's passion to push your tongue farther into their mouth. You need to follow your partner's indications to figure out when this is appropriate and desired—and when it isn't. A good rule of thumb is to feel how much of their tongue they are putting in your mouth, gently add one-fourth of an inch to that, and there's your limit. As long as you are following these signals, your kissing will be pleasurable and a delight to remember, increasing your sexual appeal and the intimacy between you. Otherwise, you may come home to a cone-shaped bra.

Also, at this level of kissing it is very important to be mindful of your breath. If you have eaten smelly food that day, it will be difficult to hide now. Remember that garlic, onions, coffee, cigarettes, and other bad-smelling consumables might make this type of kissing unpleasant for your partner. Making sure to brush, to floss, and to apply lip balm if your lips are dry and cracked are amenities your partner is sure to appreciate.

Kissing: Practice for the Big Event

Once you have practiced the exercises in this chapter for a week, and your lips are stronger, more flexible, and fully engaged, you can begin this serious tutorial of kissing techniques.

Though I wouldn't suggest trying everything in the *Kama Sutra* (there are some sections on biting and scratching your lover that seem best saved for when you're feeling über-kinky), this ancient book offers a valuable perspective on kissing that I have attempted to incorporate here. The wide diversity of kisses it recognizes points to an important insight: each kind of kiss has a specific *meaning*, and transmits something particular and distinct to your lover. Adopting this attitude toward both kissing and oral sex will enable you to read your lover's signs and signals and to respond appropriately.

Lovers are constantly sending each other messages, with every breath, every movement, and every gesture. Becoming aware of how these messages are transmitted, learning to recognize them from your partner, and sending them more clearly is the stuff of great sex. The several hundred thousand subconscious messages lovers send each other in bed (and out of bed, too!) lend sex between two individuals its distinctive character, and determine whether sex is mind-blowing or humdrum. Being aware that each of your sexual gestures sends certain messages to your partner will help you tap into the silent sensual dialogue between your bodies.

Kissing with Your Whole Self

On some level, your partner will intuitively sense your state of mind when you kiss them. They will sense your desire—and your distraction. Some people are more sensitive (or more willing to delude themselves) than others, so there will naturally be discrepancies in your lover's reception. Considering that the majority of communication is nonverbal,* and that the acts of kissing and oral sex in particular consist of a high level of physical contact in one area, it's safe to assume that you'll have trouble hiding much of anything when you're going down.

To become a great kisser, both oral and otherwise, the most important skill you can acquire is that of focus. When your lips touch your lover's skin, make sure you are fully mentally present and not just going through the motions. Do whatever it takes to focus in on the part of yourself that desires intimacy with this person. Focusing on that part will make it blossom, and will lead your eager tongue to spots divine. There is no inspiration so great as true comfort.

The following outline (roughly inspired by the *Kama Sutra*) should help you distinguish among the different types of kisses, and to become aware of all the different messages a kiss can communicate. It is set up according to levels of intensity, and while generally that progression is best (as in oral sex), it does not need to be followed to a T; rather, the best guide for what to do and when to do it is the response of your partner. Let your kissing meander and explore, returning to what works, and abandoning what doesn't without stress.

The First Kiss
For the first kiss, you might want to try a soft, tender kiss where the lips merely touch each other for a moment, without much saliva or motion, but making sure to use a little bit of the smooth inside of the

* According to Albert Mehrabian in *Nonverbal Communication* (Chicago: Aldine-Atherton, 1972). Mehrabian is credited with finding that only about 7 percent of the emotional meaning of a message is communicated through explicit verbal channels. About 38 percent is communicated by paralanguage (which is basically vocal intonation). The largest segment by far, 55 percent, comes through nonverbal communication, which includes such things as gesture, posture, and facial expression. During sex, that arena is sharply focused on the act of touching.

lip. Essentially, what this kiss says is: "I'm interested in kissing you. Care to join?" This kiss has little to do with the position of the lips, and it doesn't need any complicated hokeypokey. It transmits a simple message of interest.

If your partner responds just a little, or not at all, to this gentle kiss, you should bide your time before progressing to a more forceful kiss. Generally, the best sign that your partner is ready for an increase in intensity is their body movement. If he's moving his lips, and his hands are starting to reach for you or rub you, or his body moves closer to yours, the light doesn't get greener.

The "Relax, I'm a Great Person" Kiss

If you just made a tentative First Kiss and your partner isn't responding much, but isn't pushing you away or turning their face from you, they are probably somewhat apprehensive. This could be for a variety of reasons, personal or external. Do not rush or force this person—a few very light and nonthreatening kisses on the cheeks, forehead, and hair may open them up like a flower. Gentle conversing, good eye contact, and light embraces are the best ways to make your partner feel comfortable. These light little kisses say, "It's okay with me that you don't want to go further than this right now. I enjoy just being with you."

If correctly done, this kind of "I like just being with you" kiss will increase your sexual connection with your partner. If done with too much pressure, your partner will either feel overwhelmed or so exceptional that they will be calling you for the next millennium.

The Good Enough for Seconds Kiss

This kiss is a step beyond the first kiss, and consists of an explorative, repetitive touching of the lips that says, "Hello, here I am," then withdraws, but comes back again as if to say, "That's good enough for seconds." Picture someone tasting a new kind of ice cream cone for the first time—at first their lips touch the ice cream for a second, then they pull back, decide they like it, and go in for more. This kind of kiss can make your partner feel very special and desired. If your partner is responding well, by moving their own lips, that is the cue that they are ready for a more intense kind of kiss.

The Shower of Kisses

These are light little kisses showered all around the mouth, and can even extend to the cheeks. These kinds of kisses express how much you like your partner, as if you find their entire being wonderful and kissable, not just their lips. Again, don't move forward unless your partner is responding to your kisses with movement.

The Relationship Changer

This is a somewhat firmer kiss that clearly indicates your desire for your partner. Until now, the First Kiss, the testing kisses, and the Shower of Kisses have indicated strong liking and affection. This firmer (not forceful) return to the mouth is about more. It says, "I want you." This is the kiss that breaks platonic bonds. It is not a hard kiss, but is unquestionably somewhat stronger than the earlier ones, and uses the entire lips, as you pull one or both of their lips into yours for moments at a time.

A good way to develop this kiss at home is with a pitted plum. Choose a plum that is not too ripe or soft. Cut the plum in half and take out the pit. When you're ready, squeeze the half plum so that it shapes itself like a slightly parted mouth, and bring it to your mouth. Move your tongue beneath the top ridge of the plum, and then the bottom. Try pulling first the top edge, and then the bottom into your mouth with your lips. Use the insides of your lips to pull the ridges in. This exercise will teach you how to use your entire lips to engage your partner's mouth. As you pull in each "lip" of the plum, see if you can rhythmically suck and massage it, varying the pressure and level of suction, instead of simply pulling on it.

The Hollywood Kiss

This is the first kiss where your partner will need to open their mouth. You can try to nudge it open lightly with your mouth, but this movement should be light and gentle, not sudden or forced. If your partner opens to accept your mouth readily, let the insides of your mouths become indistinguishable and surrender to each other.

The Tongue Exploration

This kiss is not to be confused with a poke or a prod. The tongue should not be overly pointed or aggressive. Instead, the introduction of the tongue should be the silky and soft presentation of the tongue on and around the lips. Think exploration, not excavation. Simply run your tongue along and around your partner's inner lips, gently sucking their lips, one at a time, into your own mouth.

Using your tongue indicates a greater degree of intimacy between you and your partner, so be sure that your partner is comfortable with the introduction of your tongue into their mouth. Do not push your tongue past their teeth at this point. If you ever feel your partner pull away from you (even slightly), go back to something less intense.

The "I Want a Piece of You" Kiss

Once you sense your partner is getting excited and responding to your movements, you can start making your kisses firmer and deeper. The firmer you kiss your lover, the more loudly you are telling him how much you want him. Your tongue is exploring his mouth, and your hands are starting to hold him with some degree of force. Compare it to exclaiming "I want you!" right to your partner's face. In the same way that you wouldn't yell this to someone on a first date, you don't just jump straight into this kiss. It's appropriate when it is adding fuel to the fire, and not being used to ignite one.

The Love Anvil

This is a harder kiss that you give once you are 100 percent sure that your lover is so hot for you they can barely stand it. More rapid responses to your kisses, accompanied by little cries or moans, indicate that your partner's passion is hot enough to fry an egg—and that's the *only* time when it's okay to apply the Love Anvil. Use your tongue to essentially copy the rhythm of intercourse by rubbing it more passionately and with increasing speed against the taste bud side of your partner's tongue. Until now, your tongue should have stayed fairly wide, but it's okay here to point the tip a bit because the kissing has become more passionate and aggressive.

The Erotic Nibble

Now that your partner is chomping at the bit, feel free to chomp a little right back. A love bite can add sensation and eroticism to a kiss, but must be performed very carefully. Exerting control over your jaw, give your lover a little nip on the lip. Your tongue should be in the Spot for this action, because otherwise you might bite too hard or too softly. Keeping your tongue in the Spot maintains good jaw control, so that your bite can be both tender and firm. The idea here is *not* to actually hurt them, but to heighten their sensation. Before you try this with someone else, try biting the skin on your own finger first, so that you can get a sense of the strength of your jaw and the sharpness of your teeth. The Erotic Nibble is a powerful gesture; it says, "I want to consume you."

Progressing from light kisses to more intense ones—with plenty of space and time afforded for reversions, impulses, and experiments—is a good model for performing oral sex. In the same way that you would not jump right into a heavy, deeply probing kiss, oral sex requires a build-up period where your lover is given a little time to get used to the contact.

5

Oral Sex Ground Rules

YOU WILL ALWAYS have to customize oral sex for your partners: each person has a distinct set of preferences, and there's no getting around that. (We'll talk later about how to identify what those are.) But regardless of who your partner is, here are some base guidelines that lay the foundation for great oral sex.

NOT TONIGHT, HONEY . . .

The only way to truly pleasure your lover with oral sex is to approach the act with evident enthusiasm. If you don't feel like giving him oral sex, try making the atmosphere sexier and more relaxing. Focus on your favorite qualities about his physique, and move from there. Your evident, surging desire to take him in your mouth is the most important factor for a great blow job. No amount of technical skill can compensate for that. If you're truly just not in the mood, tell him how sexy he is, and promise a rain check instead of forging ahead anyway. Nothing, and I mean *nothing*, ruins good head like the feeling your partner is doing something they don't want to do.

IT AIN'T OVER TILL THE FAT LADY SINGS . . .

Do not stop giving a blow job to answer the phone or perform any activity other than another sex act. As obvious as this may seem, the number of complaints I get on this count is astonishing. You can—and should—take lingering, tantalizing pauses during oral sex to tease him like wild, and thereby increase the intensity of his eventual orgasm, but calling it quits is just plain mean. Treating your lover well means finishing what you start below the belt.

THE PRICK THAT PAINS . . .

Be careful not to use your teeth or nails on the skin of the penis with more pressure than you would use to pick up a marshmallow. If the reasoning for this isn't self-evident, you should probably have your partner sign a disclaimer before you begin.

AND THE PRICK THAT PLEASES . . .

While the penis is sensitive to sharp objects like teeth and nails, one of the greatest complaints about blow jobs (though there aren't terribly many) is that partners seem afraid to give penises firm caresses. While too much intensity is possible, it's unlikely. Also, (very) light nibbles along the shaft can be most appreciated.

NEVER UNDERESTIMATE THE POWER OF LUBRICATION

Depending on how long you want to draw it out, a really great blow job typically needs about a tablespoon of lube. Whether it's a cup of water by the bed for the lubeless, or a delicious flavored lube for the well-prepared, or even some classic K-Y, when in doubt, bring the lube out. *Always* err on the side of too much, because you're going to need more. The penis should be continually lubed, regardless of where it's going. Similarly, anything being inserted into the anus— be it a fingertip or something more creative—must be extremely well-coated in a reliable lube.

Before you apply the lube the first time, warm it by rubbing your hands together like a thoughtful masseuse. (After you've been fellating him for a while, the coolness can be refreshing, but isn't particularly welcome before.)

If you're using a condom or dental dam, put some water-based lube on the penis before it goes on to increase sensation. Don't do this if you have only oil-based lube available. Anything oil-based— and this includes lots of lubes, so make sure you read the fine print— can cause a condom to develop tiny holes.

RHYTHM NATION

Even if your technical skills aren't very honed (this shouldn't be a problem if you've been performing the exercises outlined until this point), rhythm can compensate for a lot. While taking the penis in, and almost completely out, of your mouth, you need to find the beat of your man's drum. Start by working off the rhythm that seems most pleasurable to him—be it slow and light or fast and furious—but make sure to vary your approach every once in a while.

Occasionally, you may want to take the penis entirely out of your mouth and lick it with tiny tongue strokes up and down the shaft, then put it back in and reclaim your rhythm. Later, take it out again, give a little flick lick to the head, and pop it right back in. This rhythmic variation allows the penis to become resensitized to your touch and allows for a continuing renewal of sensations. Like Thelonious Monk letting loose on the ivories, you need to throw some surprises into your beat (*without* losing your rhythm) to keep him fully interested and aroused.

LEND THAT HELPING HAND

The variety of sensations, not their source, makes or breaks a blow job. Many people make the mistake of thinking that oral sex is simply mouth sex. You really should be using your entire body to stimulate and arouse your lover. Always use your hands—and chest, and hair, and fingers—to emphasize and expand sensation while you're performing oral sex. There's no reason for the mouth to go it alone.

While it's nice when a partner can take the entire penis into their mouth, it isn't necessary when it causes discomfort. As a rule of thumb, try to take in around half the shaft, and simply use your hands to cover the rest and work with the rhythm of your mouth. Only the head requires heavy stimulation, but you should be able to move your mouth up and down the shaft a little, too. Regardless of the size of your man's member, your (well-lubed!) hands can provide a more complete sensation of immersion than your mouth alone could ever offer.

DROP THAT 'TUDE, DUDE

The next ground rule has to do with attitude. In our Western, rationalist culture, it should come as no surprise that sex is often treated as a linear progress, as in: "Partner wants orgasm. If I perform actions x, y, and z, they will result as quickly as possible in orgasm." But when has an itinerary ever made something more fun? The first step to giving truly memorable head is dropping the single-minded concern that your partner has an orgasm. Instead, try refocusing your energy on your partner's having *fun*—at every stage of the process.

YOU MUST BE CLEAN FOR SEXUAL CUISINE

A few oral sex preliminaries. In addition to your general hygiene, pay particularly close attention to the following areas: Make sure that your lips are soft and supple to the touch, and apply cocoa butter or any other moisturizer to them if they feel rough. If you plan on using your hands extensively—as you are hereby encouraged to—either make sure that your nails are clipped close to your fingers, or be hyperattentive to how and where they touch your partner's skin. And before you go down, brush those teeth. Brush 'em long and hard.

GREEN MEANS GO, RED MEANS NO, AND NOTHING MEANS...?

If your partner doesn't respond to the basic, introductory moves outlined in this book, never, ever simply proceed. Your uncertainty will affect your performance. The best thing to do in this situation is to pause and ask him how he likes it (in a confident, inviting voice). If he says he doesn't know, ask him how he feels about trying some different things, or if there is something he would like to do instead. If he's open to it, this is a great opportunity for you to experiment with different light moves, and the orgasms of a doubtful partner will make you doubly proud. However, if he responds to your question with specific directives, treat it as a learning opportunity. He may put some signature moves in your pocket.

6

The Oral Sex Fitness Test

THE TEST GETS its own chapter because you will need to keep coming back to it to check your progress. These test questions will determine whether you are ready to proceed to the next set of exercises, or if you need to keep practicing the intermediate exercises. Answer all the questions yes or no as accurately as you can; then add up the number of yeses and read the explanation after the end of the test. This is not a difficult test—wipe those images of bleary-eyed exams out of your mind. In fact, it may be the coolest test in history.

THE ORAL SEX FITNESS TEST

1. Can you make a well-defined point with your tongue? It should point straight out like an arrow, straight ahead, parallel to the ground. Try it standing in front of a mirror. Close your eyes; stick your tongue out; try and point it. Now open your eyes and check its configuration.

2. Does your tongue rest in the Spot (see chapter 3)? Your tongue has *one* correct launching pad in your mouth. Locate the Spot; then see if your tongue returns to it naturally.

3. Can you touch the corners of your mouth with the tip of your tongue—not the sides—on the first try?

4. Can you move your tongue independently of your jaw? Try this as a test: With your tongue down behind your lower teeth, pronounce a hard "k." Your jaw should open. With your tongue on the Spot and your finger between your teeth, pronounce the letters "n," "l," "t," and "d" (the letters themselves, not the sounds they make). The middle of your tongue should rub the roof of your mouth. While you're doing this, does your jaw move? Does your tongue touch your finger? They shouldn't. Stand in front of a mirror and say "cunning." If your jaw moves, you are not working your tongue independently.

5. Can you open your mouth, protrude your tongue slightly, then lift your tongue into contact with your upper lip while keeping your mouth open?

6. Can you pronounce "t," "d," "l," and "n" without touching your teeth? Can you pronounce any of the above sounds, or "h" or "s," without your tongue protruding between your teeth?

7. Can you groove your tongue?

8. Do you sleep without snoring?

9. Can you whistle with your tongue without pursing your lips?

10. Can you put your finger to the back of your mouth without gagging?

11. Do you typically avoid sore throats and colds in the winter?

12. Can you press your upper lip against your nose?

13. When you pucker your lips, are the upper and lower the same width?

14. Do you breathe while chewing?

15. Do you chew your food well before swallowing?

16. Can you eat a bowl of dry cereal without milk? Can you eat comfortably without drinking?

17. Can you speak without lisping?

18. Can you speak in any situation without stuttering?

19. Do you speak clearly, without sounding nasal?

20. Can you keep your tongue on the roof of your mouth when you are not talking?

21. Do you have good-smelling breath?

These factors each affect your ability to give great oral sex. Count your yeses and read on.

15–21: If you answered yes to more than fourteen questions, forge ahead! Your tongue has reached the level of agility it needs to perform the techniques and exercises in the next chapters.

8–14: If you answered yes to between eight and fourteen questions, you need to practice the exercises in chapter 4 for an additional nine to ten days.

0–7: If you answered yes to fewer than eight questions, stop in your tracks. You need to practice all of the exercises in the preceding chapters until you can confidently answer yes to more questions. Return to this quiz as many times as needed to measure your progress. When you're ready to move on, the exercises in chapter 7 will perfect your skills and make you a truly rare master of the mouth.

7

Basic Exercises

No member needs so great a number
of muscles as the tongue; this exceeds all the rest
in the number of its movements.

—LEONARDO DA VINCI

EXCEPT FOR THE warm-ups, each exercise you'll encounter in this chapter needs to be performed a few times a day for one to two weeks. Essentially, once your musculature is built up, oral sex itself will maintain your progress. Until you've reached that merry mixture of practice and performance, you'll need to do the exercises about once a week to avoid regressing to old (and bad) mouth habits.

Are you annoyed when people ask you to touch your tongue to your nose—because you can't? Can you tie a cherry stem in your mouth? Are you incredibly turned on by those who can? Could you touch *only* the tip of your tongue to the corners of your lips, without touching the rest of your tongue to any part of your mouth? All of these moves are oral sex assets, and if you can't do them now, these exercises will help you on your way. Rolling your tongue is a ge-netically determined trait, but the others can—and will!—be culti-vated. These movements of the tongue will be used heavily in advanced oral sex techniques, so take note. The tongue is a more complex muscle than you might think, and has a startling diversity of sensations to offer your lover. The following exercises will help you get in touch with all the possibilities.

But first things first: though you might not suspect that a tongue needs a warm-up, the kinds of techniques you will learn require a level of flexibility and suppleness that can be achieved only through a warm-up session. Skipping the warm-up can result in tongue cramps and even lockjaw, so don't skimp on these exercises because of their apparent simplicity.

- Never, ever strain yourself while performing these or any other exercises.

- The entire warm-up routine should take between five and ten minutes.

- Perform the exercise once, except where indicated.

BASIC EXERCISES

Nose Touch
Stick out your tongue and curve it up. Try to touch your nose. If you can touch your nose already, try to touch only the tip of your nose using the tip of your tongue. Repeat twice.

Chin Touch

Stick out your tongue again. Curve it down and try to touch your chin. See if you can touch your chin without the tip alone. Repeat twice.

Up and Down

Open your mouth, keeping your tongue inside and behind your teeth. Move it slowly up and down, touching the tip to the roof, then to the base. Do not run the tongue along the roof, or over the teeth. Pretend there is a toothpick between the roof of your mouth and the bottom of your jaw, and move your tongue along this perfectly vertical line. See how fast you can go while keeping the tip as the point of contact.

Side to Side

Open your mouth a little. Let your tongue peek out. Move it back and forth to each corner of your mouth on a curved path (following, but not touching, your bottom lip). Do this four times.

Peanut Butter

Open your mouth a little. Pretend you have peanut butter all over your lips. Lick all the peanut butter off your top lip, then lick it off the bottom one.

Tongue Push

Keep your lips closed. Place your tongue against one cheek and push it out, while using three fingers to gently push against the tongue from the other side of the cheek. Repeat on the other side.

Open Wide
Open and close your mouth. Letting your tongue rest on the bottom of your mouth, stretch out your cheeks but don't strain your jaw.

Smiley Face
Keeping your lips closed, give the biggest smile you can muster. Think of the oral sex master you will shortly become.

Sad Mouth
Keeping your lips closed, make the biggest frown you can.

Show Your Teeth
Keeping your teeth closed, open your lips and give a big smile. Say "extremely satisfactory" without touching your lips to your teeth.

Kisses
Pucker your lips and make one long kissing sound, keeping your lips closed, by sucking air in through your tightly contracted lips for ten seconds.

Raspberries
Keeping your lips closed and around your tongue, stick out your tongue and blow air, letting your tongue and lips vibrate. This may tickle.

Pops
Press your lips together and pop them apart, making a loud noise. Do not suck in—the popping sound is created by simply rolling your closed lips in very slightly, then allowing them to separate.

Fish Face
Push your lips out to make a fish face (*without* sucking in your cheeks for dramatic effect). Open and close your lips a few times.

Lipstick Lady
Press your lips together and rub them back and forth, as if you are spreading lipstick around on them.

Oooooh . . . Aaaaah
Focusing all of your attention on your lips, very elaborately shape your lips into the small circle that accompanies an "oooooh" sound, and hold it for about ten seconds. Then, smoothly transition into opening your mouth as far as it will go and saying "aaaaah" for ten seconds. Do each five times.

If you have successfully completed these warm-ups, congratulations! They are admittedly hard for sophisticated adults to perform.

INTERMEDIATE EXERCISES

Now that your tongue, lips, and cheeks are soft, supple, and ready to move, you're equipped to practice more advanced exercises. These exercises apply directly to oral sex, and simulate particular moves.

Tongue Cluck
Put your tongue tip behind your top teeth and get the sides of your tongue up, too. Suck in and cluck, making a horse-galloping noise.

See if you can get the middle to come down first, and the tip of the tongue last.

Focusing on getting the middle of your tongue to come down before the tip will teach your tongue how to stimulate your lover using the soft underside of the tongue instead of the rougher taste bud side. Few people know how to do this, and as the smooth side of the tongue feels delightful on the sensitive parts of the body, this exercise is well worth it!

Tsk-tsk

Use this exercise to train your tongue to use the area between the roof of your mouth and the taste bud side of your tongue to create more surrounding sensations on your lover.

With your lips open, place your tongue tip on the bump behind your top teeth and suck in gently. If you hear a sound like a disapproving old woman, you're doing it right.

Whole Tongue Suck

This exercise helps you teach your mouth to focus on a specific area, and to use sucking to heighten sensation.

With your lips slightly parted, suck your entire tongue up onto the roof of your mouth. Press and release, making a sucking sound. Repeat five times.

Tongue Stretch

This exercise will enable your tongue to reach more intricate areas, so that you can be sure to find your lover's hot spots.

Place your tongue on the roof of your mouth while you raise and lower your jaw. You should feel your tongue stretch. Repeat ten times.

Tongue Push

With your lips open, push your tongue onto the bump behind your top row of teeth for ten seconds. Relax. Repeat three times.

This is how you can learn to apply pressure with your tongue in a designated place. It will strengthen your control over when and where your tongue applies force.

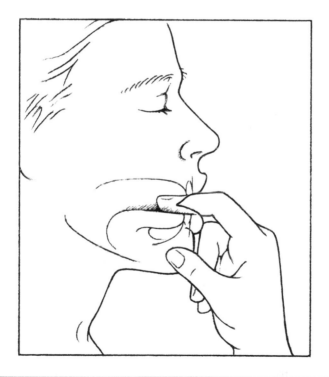

The Tongue Push

Baby Talk

Place your finger between your top and bottom rows of teeth. Practice saying these syllables: "tuh, tuh, tuh, tuh"; "duh, duh, duh, duh"; "nuh, nuh, nuh, nuh." Notice how your tongue moves down with the center first, and then the tip? Your finger should have no teeth marks on it, and should not be wet by the end of the exercise.

This will help you further develop your ability to stimulate using the soft underside of the tongue.

Crush That Candy

Take a small piece of circular candy (the size of a Skittle or M&M). Use your tongue to press the candy into the bump behind your front row of teeth, but not touching it. Press the candy with your tongue steadily, until it breaks or dissolves. Do not repeat. For the health conscious, a Cheerio works exceptionally well.

This exercise tones and strengthens the tongue and, if practiced regularly, will eliminate fatigue.

KKK (Not That One)

Keeping your tongue tip down behind your lower teeth, open your mouth and make a "k-k-k" sound by lifting the back of your tongue.

When your lover is ready for more intense stimulation, use this tongue motion to stimulate them with the rough, taste bud side of your tongue.

More Imaginary Peanut Butter

Pretend you have peanut butter all over your bottom lip. Stretch your top lip over your bottom lip and pretend to wipe all the peanut butter off, addressing the sides as well as the front.

For supersensitive areas on your lover, the lip is a great substitution for the tongue. The soft inside of the upper lip can extend in the manner exercised to caress and awaken sensitive spots that can be stimulated more aggressively with the tongue later.

Hold It and Blow

Practice blowing a cotton ball across a table by using just a straw held firmly between your lips. In doing this, focus on learning how to apply specific amounts of pressure with the air you exert from your mouth. This will both fine-tune the muscles of your mouth and teach your tongue to flatten at just the tip—an excellent position from which to initiate upward strokes over the head of the penis (or other supersensitive areas) with definite feeling but not an overwhelming degree of it.

Different Strokes

Pretend that you have whipped cream all over the roof of your mouth. Using the tip of your tongue, sweep it from front to back along the roof of your mouth. Do this for ten strokes, then change direction, noting the difference in sensation.

The basic exercises in this chapter should be performed religiously for the first one to two weeks, but you can relax them somewhat and focus on the intermediate exercises for an additional week. (This is because the intermediate exercises build off of and hone the raw skills developed by the warm-ups.) Take the Oral Sex Fitness Test in chapter 6 to make sure that you're ready to move on, because the exercises beyond this point are intended for advanced practitioners only.

8

Quitters Never Climax:
Breathing for Oral Sex

ND YOU THOUGHT it was just "through the nose." If you've ever run out of breath, or suddenly needed to stop during oral sex, this chapter is especially for you. Instead of gagging, running out of energy, or feeling like you've been on a three-day expedition to Mt. Orgasm, you can learn to breathe and control the muscles of your lips and mouth in a way that will keep you happy, comfortable, and energized for truly boundless oral sex.

Just because you can breathe well enough to keep yourself alive doesn't mean you're doing it correctly. Imagine someone hopping into a race car and joining a competition just because they have a standard-issue driver's license. Well, our bodies are equally complex and powerful, and it takes skill and know-how to handle them for peak performance. And unfortunately, most of us are treating our bodies like rent-a-wrecks.

PUT A TIGER IN YOUR TANK

Breathing properly is the fastest and most efficient source of energy available to a human being. Putting oxygen in your lungs keeps you alert, vigorous, and ready for physical activity. Unfortunately, it isn't as easy as it seems to pull air directly into your lungs. The only way to really get the air to come swiftly and directly into your lungs— rather than your stomach—is to breathe in through your nose with your lips closed, and that's not a habit most of us have truly acquired. Think about it this way: If you put food in your mouth, it goes into your stomach. Well, the same goes for air. Trying to breathe by putting air in your mouth is about as effective as trying to eat by putting food up your nose. Sure, a little bit will make it down there. But you need more than a little, especially when you're hard at work giving a good *mange*.

As for oral sex, there are several reasons that you should learn to breathe correctly. In order to perform oral sex for any significant period of time, you need to be able to pull lots of fresh oxygen in your lungs quickly and easily, without gasping or gulping. Have you ever been giving someone oral sex, and felt kind of like you were doing a bunch of work for nothing? You may give all sorts of interpretations to thoughts like these, but they're simple and natural responses to an insufficient oxygen supply to your muscles. Proper breathing can keep that oxygen flowing into the active muscles, which will keep you feeling good about giving your partner pleasure with plenty of extra energy to go on a riff when you get inspired.

The rest of this chapter presents a quick and dirty regime to help you gain control and mastery over your breathing. It's basically divided into two parts, with two objectives. The first segment is made up of exercises to help you relax the throat and jaw muscles, and will make your lips, tongue, and neck more flexible and less likely to cramp. The second will help you to develop better involuntary breathing habits, and will help your stamina and overall performance.

THROAT AND JAW BREATHING EXERCISES

Tension in the throat and jaw area is one of the most restricting factors to pleasurable oral sex performance. If your throat and jaw muscles are too tight, your flexibility and comfort will be compromised. These exercises will also help you develop a pleasant, powerful speaking voice.

Head Rolls
To relax the throat and jaw muscles, sit in a chair or on the floor with your back straight and supported by a wall. Make sure the surface is hard enough to support a straight back, no matter what posture your head might be in. A good way to test this is to find a place where you can sit comfortably, then move your head in a circle. If your spine collapses forward, you're not using a firm enough surface. Make sure you choose a spot where you can move your head in a circle without significant movement in your spine.

Once you're situated, relax your shoulders and let your head begin to roll to the right across your chest *without* exerting any energy. Imagine your head is a big balloon filled with water, and you are simply letting it roll forward. Exhale while your head rolls across the chest in a clockwise circle, and inhale as it starts to roll across your shoulders. Feel the tension draining out of your neck and jaw. *Don't* try to stretch or strain yourself. No pressing, and no pulling. If you feel strain anywhere, restrict your motion to a smaller circle. Now reverse the direction, rolling your head counterclockwise. Keep alternating direction every two or three revolutions, exhaling and letting your mouth open as your head comes back, inhaling and letting your mouth close as you roll your head forward.

Once you've started to relax the muscles of your neck and throat (about one minute), allow your tongue to swell and grow heavy in your mouth as you're rolling. You can even stick it out a little and let it come between your teeth. Allow your tongue to be so big and heavy that it can roll in the direction of your head. Practice for two or three minutes, three times a day.

This throat and jaw relaxing exercise is great because of its versatility—you can do it for a moment while sitting at your desk, waiting in the doctor's office, or even at a red light. The more you do it, the happier your throat and jaw muscles will be, and the less likely they will be to give up on you or wear out during oral sex.

TENSING AND RELAXING

This second segment of breathing exercises is a more systematic way to relax your neck, throat, and jaw muscles. If you have never practiced exercises like the one in this book before, you should do the Head Rolls first before moving on to this.

These exercises may seem simple, but they can have a great effect on the state of these muscle groups, so they need to be practiced with care and caution. It is very easy to throw these muscle groups out of balance—I should know, because I've spent my whole life correcting them! So move forward gently, and don't start practicing *any* exercise too suddenly or vigorously. Remember: going slow and gently during the exercises will help you to be vigorous and energized in bed, but doing the exercises slapdash and at breakneck speed will only hurt your performance.

Find a spot where your spine is fully supported, and where you can bend your head forward without causing your spine to bend forward, too. Sit with your spine as straight as possible. The idea behind this exercise is very simple and very powerful: creating tension within certain muscles, and then releasing that tension. Most people are constantly storing their stress in the muscle groups of their neck and jaw area. When you consciously put tension into these muscles and then relax them, it gathers up all the other tension you stored in these muscles during your day at work and flushes it out, too.

For the next few minutes, you will be taking deep breaths in through your nose with your lips closed, tensing up a particular group of muscles for a certain amount of time. Then, with your tongue tip down, and mouth relaxed and open, you will exhale and release all the tension in those muscles while the air is flowing out. The most important elements are taking a deep enough breath—inhale slowly enough to fill your entire lungs—and knowing exactly which muscle groups to tense. This will entirely fill your lungs with fresh air—a rare treat for them.

Releasing Closed-Mouth Tension

In this first exercise, we'll create closed-jaw tension. With your tongue on the Spot (see page 30), take a deep breath through your nose, hold it, and close your mouth tightly at the same time. Press your lips together tightly, press your molars together tightly, and press your tongue into the Spot like there's no tomorrow. Tense the muscles slowly but surely in the span of about five seconds, until they are as hard as rocks and as tense as they can possibly become. Hold for a count of ten, pressing with an extra push for the last count.

Now, let it go! As the air flows out of your lungs, all of the tension will drain out of your lips, jaw, and mouth. Take a few breaths here, concentrating on how relaxed those muscles are, now that their tension has been drained from them. Give your head a little shake, allowing your face to shake like a rag doll, to release any leftover tension. Repeat, making sure to *let the air and the tension flow out of your mouth at the same time.*

Releasing Open-Mouth Tension
For this next tense-and-relax exercise, we'll create and release open-mouth tension. Be very careful with this exercise—do not do it if you have any pain in your jaw.

After you inhale with your tongue on the Spot, open your mouth fairly widely until you feel the tension in the jaw hinge. Depending on the shape of your mouth, your tongue may want to come off the Spot, which is fine. As you're opening your mouth, stretch your lips forward as far as they will go. Increase the tension slowly, but don't open so wide that you feel any kind of pain. Hold for a count of five, giving a little extra push at the last count, and then let go of the air in your lungs and the tension in your face at the same time. Close your mouth as the stress flows away with the air.

Repeat, again opening your mouth fairly widely, and stretching your lips out as far as they will go. You may look a little like Mr. Ed getting ready for his feeding, but the overall effect on your jaw muscles is tremendous. Yawning is a natural response to this posture—just let it happen, shake it out, and start over.

Take a couple of breaths before you do this next one, enjoying the sensation of relaxed muscles in your neck and jaw. This time, with your tongue on the Spot, inhale through your nose and start to stretch out your lips again. But this time, point your chin straight up as well. Feel a gentle stretching or a pulling being generated along your throat from the tip of your chin to about halfway down the length of your throat. Again, increase the stretch slowly without going to the point of pain. Hold your breath and stretch it out for a count of five, and then exhale your chin back to neutral and let the tension in your throat and lips flow out at the same time.

This time, you're going to put your tongue in the Spot, inhale, and lean your head forward and down to your chest. Press your chin firmly against your chest and feel the tension building in the front of your throat as you hold the air in your lungs. Build the pressure slowly, and again, back off before you reach the point of pain. Keep your chin pressed down, the air in your lungs, and stretch for a count of five. Let the tension spill out with the exhale. Repeat.

Releasing Upper-Body Tension
As you inhale with your tongue on the Spot, close your eyes, press your lips together, bring your elbows tightly into your ribs, and hold your throat in a swallowing position. That's inhale, lips closed, eyes closed, elbows pulled in, and—swallow! Hold for a count of three and let it go. Let the air out slowly, and the tension in those muscles should exit slowly with the exhaled air. Breathe in and out for a moment, just feeling the new absence of tension in those muscles. Repeat.

At this point, close your eyes and scan the head, neck, and upper body for areas where you personally might be storing excess tension. Do you remember a massage or physical therapist mentioning that there's a certain place where you tend to store tension? Those areas would be a great place to start. You should now take a moment to isolate those muscles and release their tension. Perhaps you tend to store tension in your shoulders—you can lift them up or pull them back and then release. Or maybe it's your stomach, in which case you can push out on the abdominal wall and then release. Choose whatever muscle group you feel could use a little relaxing.

Once you've identified an area where you're storing tension, inhale with your tongue on the Spot, hold your breath, and tense those muscles as tight as they will go without causing you pain. Hold and press for a count of three, then allow the air to leave your lungs, and let it carry out the tension with it. Repeat. Feeling and enjoying the release that takes place after each exercise is just as important as performing the exercises themselves, so take a moment between each one to appreciate the absence of tension in whatever muscle group you've worked on.

Remember:

- Be careful whenever you exert tension into a push or a stretch. Build the pressure slowly, and never take it to the point of pain.

- Do these exercises with the written description to guide you for the first couple of days, but after that, feel free to practice them in the office, on the subway, or even in the shower.

- You will need to do these exercises two or three times a day for several days before you're ready to move on to the more advanced breathing and muscle-relaxing exercises.

DEVELOPING A RELAXATION REFLEX

Now that you've gone through and systematically tensed and released the muscles in your neck, throat, and jaw for several days, you should be getting more and more conscious of the presence or absence of tension in these muscle groups. You should also be creating an association in your mind—and in your body—between the release of a deep breath and the release of physical stress. If that association becomes strong enough, you should become increasingly able to consciously trigger a relaxation reflex in the muscle groups you have worked with. This will prove to be incredibly helpful during oral sex.

If you regularly perform these breathing exercises, you will never have lockjaw or painful lips and muscles during oral sex again.

Let's do a little test to see if the relaxation reflex has already begun to be established in your mind and body. Sit with your back straight and let your mind go back to the time when you were performing the tensing-and-relaxing exercises. Visualize yourself taking a deep breath, tensing your muscle groups, holding, and finally letting those muscle groups release their tension with the air in your lungs. Now prepare yourself to take a deep breath *without* tensing up any of your muscles. This time, when you have taken a deep breath with your tongue on the Spot and are holding the air in your lungs, use the time to allow your mind to simply scan your body for any tension. Concentrate on this tension so that when you exhale, you can let it spill out with the air. Feel the relaxation this inspires and repeat four more times. Scan your body for pockets of tension, and keep performing these exercises until there aren't any left. Simply performing them will teach your muscles to relax in response to internalized stress.

Now that you've reached this point, don't leave Head Rolls and the tensing-and-relaxing exercises in the dust. Keep doing these exercises at least twice a day—they are positively wonderful for your mind and upper body, as well as for your respiratory system. But, in addition, two or three times during the day practice your relaxation reflex. This will be marvelous for your overall health and stamina. If you're walking into a high-pressure meeting, or sitting down to dine with a first date, the relaxation reflex will help you be your calmest, most centered, and charming self.

Remember:

- When you're practicing the relaxation reflex, try to feel every ounce of tension flowing out of your upper body.

- It's extremely important to relax these muscles before performing the kind of strenuous oral sex that this guide will inspire you to.

- Always, always, always breathe in through your nose during these exercises, and keep your tongue on the Spot during the inhalations. If the tongue is down, it will block the air passageway and prevent the lungs from filling completely with air.

Although at first glance breathing may seem unrelated to oral sex, poor breathing is actually what makes oral sex uncomfortable for most people. When you're breathing correctly, you can soften and energize your face, neck, and lips muscles to an extent otherwise impossible to give limitless pleasure to your lover.

9

Serious Sexercises

THE REALLY CRUCIAL tongue exercises may be fewer in number than the exercises in preceding chapters, but they are the most potent exercises in the book. So if you're short on time and patience, this is where you should focus your attention. While most of the exercises until now have been fairly specialized, focusing on certain moves, techniques, and parts of the tongue and lips, these exercises are the quick-and-dirty guide to getting maximum strength and flexibility out of your tongue.

Boyfriend's Delight

This exercise is designed to train your tongue to rest in the most energizing position possible. The correct positioning of the tongue will also help you to get maximum flexibility and range in the lips. Place a Cheerio on the bump behind your top row of teeth. Keep it in place by pressing with your tongue. Now swallow, *without* moving the Cheerio. You will need to significantly increase the pressure of your tongue to stop the Cheerio from moving, thus building the strength and correcting the orientation of your tongue. (You'll know you're done with each Cheerio when it begins to become soft.)

This exercise is so fundamental to developing an agile, capable tongue that ideally you should go through a whole bowl of Cheerios. Barring that, try ten to fifteen. Try to keep your tongue in the same position for increasing periods of time—ideally, in fact, your tongue should always be in this position, with your lips closed and breathing through your nose.

If you have trouble breathing through your nose, and often forget to keep your lips closed, try resting a twist tie (or toothpick, or plastic paper clip, or any small, lightweight item) between your lips. This gives your lips a "reason" to close, and if it falls out, you'll be alerted that your lips are open. In this way, you can become more aware of the state of your lips and their relationship to your breathing.

To supplement this exercise after you've practiced it a few times, try to swallow every time with your tongue in that exact spot—regardless of what drink fills your glass or food fills your plate. These swallows are like push-ups for your tongue, and they're healthy for your whole mouth. The next time you go to give oral sex, you will be just as delighted as your partner is to see how masterfully you can create specific sensations.

Boyfriend's Double Delight

This is essentially like Boyfriend's Delight, except this time you are going to use two Cheerios: one placed on the bump behind your top row of teeth, and the other placed about a half inch beyond that, toward your throat. This will activate more of your tongue by getting the midsection to keep the second Cheerio in place during the swallow.

Once again, extend your practicing this exercise into each mealtime: every time you swallow, try to do it this way. It will help your digestion as much as your oral sex skills. But don't swallow the Cheerios—the object is to keep them precisely in place.

Yet Another "Delight"
That's right: add one more Cheerio. Place the third Cheerio another half inch beyond the second one. Just do the three-Cheerio swallow a couple of times to see if you can. If it's too difficult, that means you need to practice the earlier Delights. If it's easy, move on to the next exercise.

It's Time Again: Checkpoint
It can't be overemphasized how important a well-defined point is to oral sex, so go to the mirror for this one and make a mental note of what follows. Stick your tongue straight out as far as it will go, and bring the tip to the sharpest point you can make. Repeat three times.

As you do this exercise, check whether your tongue is changing color. If it was grayish or whitish, the Cheerio exercises should be making it pinkish, the natural color of a healthy, vigorous tongue. Is your tongue rather bulbous instead of coming to a well-defined point? Does the tip, when extended, point either to the left or right of center? You should give special attention to this exercise until your tongue makes a well-defined point and these symptoms of a poorly pointed tongue disappear.

Open and Close
Open your mouth as wide as possible and stick out your tongue as far as it will go. Make your tongue long and pointed at the tip, then draw it in slightly to shorten and widen it as wide as it will go. Repeat this five times.

Oral Play

This exercise will give dexterity to your tongue, enable you to use the tip accurately, and employ a well-defined point.

Hold your lower jaw down with thumb and forefinger. Touch the tip of your tongue to the upper right molar, then the upper left molar, lower left molar, lower right molar, in that order. Raise your tongue to the Spot (see page 30). Lower the tip of your tongue to the roots of your lower front teeth. Repeat six times.

Open Your Jaw

Curl up your tongue and place it as far back on the roof of your mouth as possible. With your tongue locked in that position, open and close your mouth. Repeat fifteen times. This exercise will reteach you how to have control over the movement of your jaws and eliminate involuntary movement.

Getting in the Groove

Stick out your tongue. Now groove it. Bring it back into your mouth. If you're having trouble, use a straw to roll the sides of your tongue on. Repeat ten times.

Keep in mind that a groove (pulling the center of the tongue down below the bottom row of teeth) is unlike a roll (where the sides of the tongue roll together). Grooving the tongue, unlike rolling it, is not genetically determined and can be accomplished with a little practice by virtually anyone.

Rolling Around

Place the tip of your tongue down behind your lower front teeth with your mouth open. Make sure it is touching the teeth right at their roots. Hum so the center of your tongue touches the palate.

With the tongue in this position, rotate it from right to left. Repeat five times. Watch in the mirror to make sure your jaw doesn't move.

This exercise will straighten and firm the muscles in the center of the tongue.

Weight Lifting

Place the handle of a spoon on the center of your tongue. Keeping the spoon steady, push upward with the tongue and hold for a count of three. Relax the tongue, and then repeat four times. Do this three times a day. As you become proficient in this exercise, try to keep the tongue back in the mouth, perhaps just over the front teeth. This is the kind of weight lifting your boyfriend dreams of.

If you've completed these exercises, your tongue is the most agile, strong, and delicate it's ever been, capable of quickly transitioning between feathery love tickles and intense, aggressive stroking before he has time to say "aah." But now that you have such a big strong tongue, what *are* you going to do with it?

10

Becoming a Fellatrix

The way to a man's heart is through his . . .

IF YOU SAID "stomach," you haven't been paying very close attention. Let's get one thing straight: even mediocre blow jobs make men happy. Unlike with a woman's vagina, where you can't always count on lingual caresses to translate into pleasurable sensations, simply taking his penis into your mouth is going to make your man feel pretty swell. Barring the presence of a scraping tooth, it's downright difficult to take the pleasure out of a blow job.

But if it's hard to give a completely unsatisfying blow job, it's equally hard to give a truly spectacular one. Precisely because they can make their partner climax without having to learn or develop skills, most people never treat him to the vast range of sensations oral sex can offer. And the majority of men, having never experienced these outer reaches, are hardly the best judges of their partners. As long as there are still people who think blow jobs are gross, or undignified, or who simply won't give them (and believe me, there're plenty of these), the bar is going to remain relatively low on BJ performance.

So if our men already act like they've won the lottery every time we get them off, why should we even try to improve our skills? Aren't we already doing them a favor by giving a blow job in the first place?

While it's true that you can please your man by simply forming your mouth into an O and bobbing juicily up and down for a while, the moaning, head-tossing, mattress-slapping, I-think-I-might-be-dying-but-please-don't-stop *whoppers* require more sophisticated tactics. Think more Fred Astaire than *Stomp!* To get the kinds of orgasms that will leave your man cross-eyed, a few up-and-down gestures and a little head play isn't going to do the trick. There are guidelines to follow, body parts to learn, and specific oral techniques to acquire.

Giving oral sex becomes more fun in direct proportion to the amount of pleasure it creates—the more you can unravel his sanity with the slightest touch of your tongue, the more fun you'll have below his belt. So let's hop to it!

11

Getting to Know Him Below the Belt:
An Anatomy Lesson You'll Like

YOU WOULD BE surprised at the number of people—wives, girlfriends, and one-night stands alike—who refuse to even *look* for a prolonged period at a penis, much less suck one until a man is in a state of blinding ecstasy. Some women who have been married for twenty years or more can't describe the different parts of the penis, while others aren't even aware that the penis *has* distinct features because they don't like to touch their partner's penis with their hands.

Like everything else, nature has marked the human penis with a love of variety. The penis can range in color from a creamy, cherry-blossom pink to a dark-chocolate brown, and its shape is hardly democratic. Ranging from less than three to more than thirteen inches, the penis can narrow to a fine point, widen from its base, or lay as level as a piece of timber. The only guarantee is that your man's penis will be entirely unique. Its shape, by the way, is no indication of how it will feel inside you—sometimes that funny curve is just enough to hit your G-spot, while a ramrod might leave you unexpectedly wanting more. Beyond the visuals, penises are as different in likes and dislikes as the men they're attached to.

But unlike many men, penises will immediately tell you what they're feeling. If they like something, they grow bigger. If they don't, they shrink. For this reason, you need to form a personal bond with your man's most expressive organ. It will reveal more secrets to you about giving him head than anything else.

To kick off this mutually rewarding relationship, the first thing you need to do is to really *look* at your partner's penis—and not just a cursory glance or a horrified, furtive survey. If you're not sure how this will make your partner feel, simply suggest that some kind of reward is in store for him if he lets you gaze at "length."

When you first pull the penis out for your inspection, it will most likely be flaccid. But it probably won't take long for a full erection to blossom under your gaze. Ideally, you should both be nude; you don't want to make him feel that he's in the doctor's office (unless of course you're playing the nubile nurse).

MASCULINE ANATOMY: LET'S HANG OUT

The male penis is a fairly complex and intricate organ, despite its apparent simplicity. It is extremely distinct from the rest of the male body, complete with a unique type of skin. While most of us would have no trouble identifying the differences between a circumcised and uncircumcised penis, understanding the wide range of more subtle distinctions requires a bit more study.

Aside from the *shaft*, the *meatus* (the opening in the head of the penis to allow ejaculate to come out), and the *head*, which are fairly self-explanatory, there are two distinct areas of the penis that are of particular importance to oral sex:

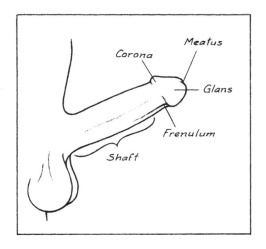

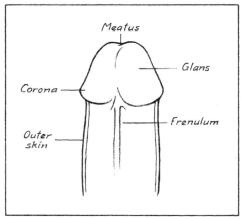

The Circumcised Penis

- The reddish or purplish *glans* or *glans penis* (head of the penis that begins above the ridge) is smooth, shiny, moist and extremely sensitive.

- The *frenulum*, or *frenum*, is a connecting membrane on the underside of the penis, similar to that beneath the tongue.

Of the various parts of the penis, the all-important anatomy for oral sex on a circumcised man is the *frenulum* and the *glans*. For an uncircumcised man, add to this the *foreskin* and the *frenar band*. Each of these structures creates a different feeling when stimulated, and each contributes a vital aspect to a man's experience of oral sex.

The Shaft
In a young or inexperienced partner, you may find that shaft stimulation alone creates an orgasm rather quickly—as will perhaps the sight of nude breasts. On an older or more experienced partner, don't waste your time. Your man will love it if you make his sensations more complete by encircling his shaft in your hands and moving them rhythmically with your mouth as you fellate him, but letting the shaft take center stage is for times when you want to slow things down, since it is not nearly as dense in nerve endings as the other parts of the penis.

The Glorious Glans
You will notice that at the top of the shaft there is a bulbous part of the penis usually called the head. This is the largest concentration of nerve endings in the penis, making the glans extremely responsive to stimulation—and sometimes (especially after orgasm) even painfully sensitive to the touch.

The outer perimeter of the glans is called the *corona*, which joins the head to the shaft. This little ridge is the more specific spot where the main nerve endings of the glans are concentrated. This ridge loves to be approached from both above and below. Since most men are more sensitive on one side than the other, try both on a new partner and pay close attention to the moans or bodily spasms stimulating each side elicits.

The levels of stimulation good for the glans will vary during the pleasure cycle, so keep a watchful eye out for signals to turn up the volume, to keep it right there, or to lay off for a while.

Engaging the glans when a full erection is already in place will raise the intensity level from hot to orgasmic. Until you're ready for that shift, light licking and sucking is more than enough to grace the glans, an area powerful enough to trigger an orgasm all by itself. The bottom line? Go wild on the glans when you're ready for him to climax.

If your man is uncircumcised, a great way to lightly engage the glans while he's still soft is by poking your tongue inside the space between the foreskin and the glans beneath. Poking and prying into this very sensitive area creates a variety of tantalizing sensations, which are heightened even more by the introduction of an ice cube or a mouthful of warm water.

The Fantastic Frenulum

Once there's a well-developed erection, the skin of the frenulum (and frenar band, if he has one) is stretched tightly enough from the corona to become extremely responsive to the lightest lick of your warm, wet tongue. As always, make sure that your tongue is very moist and exploratory. Licking and sucking the frenulum and the frenar band is another move that heightens the intensity of his sensations, and will create an orgasmic state very quickly.

If you follow the ridge of the corona around to the underside of the penis (in most positions, this should be the side facing you), you'll notice a point where the two ends of the corona come together. If your partner is uncircumcised, this will also be the place where the foreskin is attached, making it a junction of extraordinary pleasure. Frequently referred to as the "sweet spot," this tiny area is easily the most sensitive one on the entire male body, the closest a man will ever get to the compacted sensitivity of a clitoris. The location can vary from just below the meatus to the circumcision scar.

On uncircumcised men, the frenar band essentially consists of a series of ridges, and sensations from these structures during arousal are thought to be the primary trigger of orgasm in the adult male (while *Sports Illustrated*'s swimsuit issue is perhaps the primary orgasmic trigger of the adolescent male). These ridges are loaded with Meissner's corpuscles, and thus respond very readily to pressure, loading his entire lower body with rippling sensations of driving, building, and even excruciating pleasure. Handle with care, because once you start messing around with the frenar band, your baby's gonna blow. (For more information on the exact location of the frenar band, turn to page 96.)

Circumcision's Circumstances

All circumcised men have a scar on the shaft of the penis. Its location varies—sometimes it is closer to the head, while other times it appears further down the shaft. Make sure to identify the location of this scar and to lightly test a caress there before you begin performing oral sex. In some men, the scar becomes very tender and even painful to the touch. If your partner has a loss of feeling due to circumcision, supplement your oral sex by stimulating other sensitive areas.

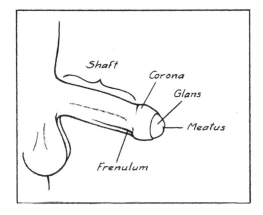

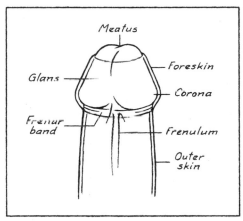

The Uncircumcised Penis

Them That's Got: The Uncircumcised Penis

An uncircumcised partner has the advantage of several additional (and extremely sensitive) parts to play with. They are:

- The *outer foreskin layer,* a continuation of the skin of the shaft of the penis.

- The *inner foreskin layer,* which is not really "skin," but mucocutaneous tissue of a unique type found nowhere else on the body.

- The *frenar band* is the interface (join) between the outer and inner foreskin layers. When the penis is not erect, it tightens to narrow the foreskin opening. During erection, the frenar band forms a ridge that goes all the way around, about halfway down the shaft.

The Friendly Foreskin

The foreskin is particularly helpful during early stages of arousal, as stimulating it helps to trigger an erection. Chock-full of nerve receptors easily stimulated by stretching, and by being rubbed over the surface of the glans, the foreskin can make pleasure ricochet through your lover's body. A unique and fine piece of bodywork, the foreskin contains special sensory receptors called Meissner's corpuscles, which scientists believe are specially designed to provide pleasure. Don't worry about pronouncing it; just use them for all they're worth.

Testy Testicles

The testicles are sensitive, temperamental creatures. Hanging softly and quietly beneath the shaft, you wouldn't spot them as troublemakers right away. But grabbing them or handling them at all roughly creates a kind of agony the "second sex" may never know.

Running your fingers very lightly on the undersides of the testicles while you fellate your partner—and using your fingertips, not your nails—may add an exciting lift to his orgasm, or it may detract from the experience. It all depends on his unique makeup. On this count, it's best to follow your partner completely. After all, who could be a better guide to handling the family jewels than someone who's been polishing them all his life?

Lightly stimulating the testicles after the erection is launched, but well before ejaculation, is a great way to find out where the testicles register on your man's pleasure/pain scale. If gently stroking them with your fingers elicits a soft moan, obviously you're in the clear. But if he gets quiet and a little stiff, as if trying to determine exactly how much you're going to insist on touching him there, leave those grouchy gonads behind and don't turn back.

If you find out that he's a DSMT (Don't Stroke My Testicles), feel free to try the perineum behind the testicles. This area, described below, is equally responsive to light caresses but is, generally speaking, much more easygoing.

"Sucking the tea bag" is when a partner very delicately takes one or both of the testicles wholly into their mouth. Humming while you have them in can produce a surprisingly pleasant sensation, as can a small chip of ice or mouthful of warm water introduced just before the "tea bags." For more information on this technique, turn to page 136.

What Up, G?

The prostate, which is sometimes called the "male G-spot," unleashes wildly erotic possibilities and orgasms unsurpassed if you're willing to go on a little dig. About the size of a condom, the prostate is located about three inches into the anal canal toward the penis. When he's aroused, this point will swell and become firm, and may be easier to locate. This area is directly connected to erectile impulses, making it a great place to get started, too.

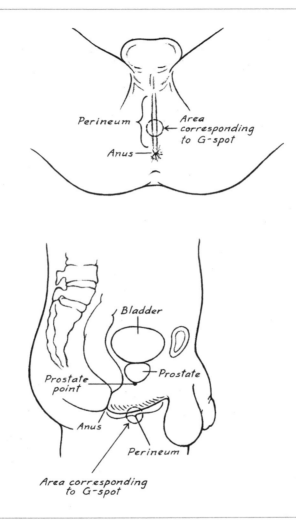

Finding the Male G-spot

Another important G-location is the "prostate point," which can be reached by pressing a finger one-third of the way from the anus toward the testicles, on the perineum. This point can provide excellent heightened sensations for those who are feeling a little timid about anal insertion.

To reach the "promised land," slowly (at a snail's pace) insert a warm, well-lubed finger (or sex toy) into his anus while you're fellating him. Give him a moment to adjust, and once you're in to the second knuckle, ever so gently begin to make a repeated "come hither" motion with your finger. This movement will make the tip of your finger tap his G-spot. This is his magic lantern, so rub yourself silly.

This may produce an explosive orgasm on contact, so be prepared. If it produces no response, start wider and move in a circle until you hit the prostate. The first third of the skin leading from the rectum to the prostate is the most sensitive area. Having his prostate stimulated in this fashion can incite some of the most powerful orgasms a man can experience. The enormous amount of nerve transference to the area makes it possible for men to have such orgasms from prostate stimulation alone.

The Miracles of Middle Earth

Behind the balls and between the thighs is a stretch of skin that is a fantastic gift to everyone involved. Responsive to stimulation, but never hypersensitive like the glans or testicles, this area is technically called the *perineum*, but deserves some finer name. It is the BJ giver's ace in the hole.

Beneath the skin of the perenium is where the bulb of the penis (its "root") is located, and when the penis becomes erect this area also hardens. No matter what stage of the pleasure cycle you've reached, stroking and rubbing this area will probably make it better. Many men find it particularly pleasurable to have this area lightly stroked with a back-to-front motion (with the finger pads or the tips

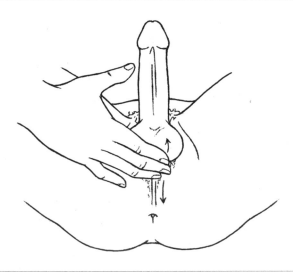

Stroking the Perineum

of the nails) that also pulls the balls ever so slightly forward while being fellated.

In the other direction, the prostate point is also located on the
perenium, about two-thirds of the way back near the outside of the
anus. Remember that this is your G-spot connection, so a light massage, circular rubbing, or even simple rhythmic tapping is of particular value here.

Don't Be an Ignoranus

An area of stimulation for many men—though not all—is the anus.
Some men will lose their load immediately when you lightly blow
on or caress the anus during oral sex; others are less responsive or
have difficulty receiving pleasure in a "taboo" spot. If you want to
do more than lightly blow and tickle, it's very easy to use a dental

dam or cut open a condom (unroll and cut up one side, removing the curved tip to create a flat, large square) to make oral stimulation of the anus safer. Especially if you don't know your partner very well, make sure that you take some sort of precaution, because hepatitis A and E can be transmitted through anal contact.

If your man doesn't want the full insertion of a G-spot search, but is open to something a little less intense, barely entering this tight sphincter with your tongue (through a dam) or well-lubed fingertip can create fantastic sensations, and will heighten his orgasms considerably. However, rimming isn't usually enough on its own to bring a man to a full, satisfying climax.

OTHER EROGENOUS ZONES

Whenever possible, include nearby—and not so nearby—body parts in your oral sex. Limiting oral sex to genitalia is like tethering a stallion. You want your man to have all-over orgasms that encompass him entirely and send waves of pleasure rolling through his entire body. This cannot be achieved by isolating the genitals. Your stimulation has to be multifarious, diffuse. In a word, get those damn hands out there! Pinch and play, stroke and tickle, rub and caress the orgasm into every part of his body.

Nipples
Many men are extremely sensitive to the licking, caressing, sucking, and pinching of their nipples—even if some of them aren't yet even aware of it. One time, I went a little wild on a new partner's nipple, and he climaxed simply from surprise and excitement. Don't forget that the nipples are sitting there packed with nerve endings, and they

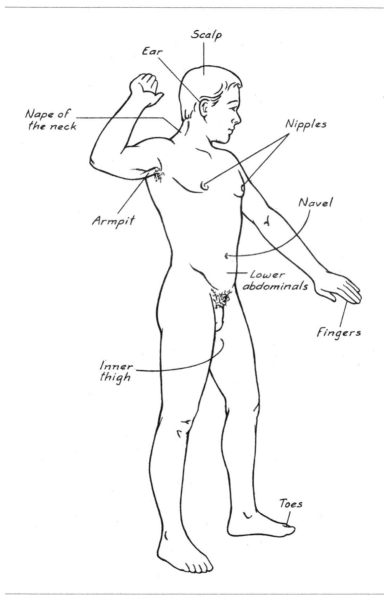

All-over Erogenous Zones

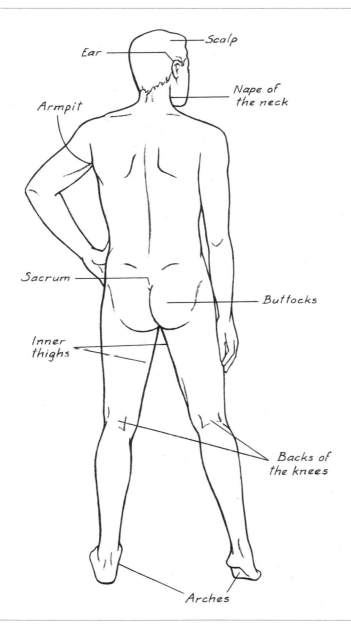

Scalp

Ear

Nape of
the neck

Armpit

Sacrum

Buttocks

Inner
thighs

Backs of
the knees

Arches

All-over Erogenous Zones

love to be played with. Also, many men like to have their nipples pinched or pulled in a way that would be painful to a woman. Don't let your own sensitive breasts stop you from clamping on.

Ears

The ears are nerve hothouses. You can lick them, suck them, stroke them, and lovingly nibble or lightly bite them. The only ear rule is to avoid breathing too hard into the ear canal. You want to express your enthusiasm, but making noises like a huffing Doberman isn't the best way to do it.

The Butt

The cheeks of the butt on both men and women have an automatic sexual response linked to them, which is strengthened by repeated pressure.

A firmly pressured butt cheek massage, or simply moving your palms over them in slow, deep circles during oral sex, can really get the sex juices flowing. So can really rhythmic pressure of any kind on this area. Spanking, if your partner is into it, also releases all kinds of sexual hormones into the bloodstream that will give a kick to your "bad boy."

Backs of the Knees

These deserve a lot more credit and attention than they usually get. An extremely sensitive area, the crevices where the skin comes together behind the knees is a great place for teasing and foreplay. Also, if your man is lying down, you can have him prop his knees up and gently tickle him with one hand behind the knees while fellating him with your mouth and the other hand. The only trick is that the skin needs to be soft and dry—so use this technique early on, before your bodies are too sleek with sweat.

The Neck

The neck is made of soft and very delicate skin that loves to be lightly stroked and kissed. Whenever you think of it, reach up there and run your fingers along the nape of his neck.

Scalp

The scalp doesn't get half the attention it deserves. Plenty of people remember that this is a sensitive spot during foreplay, when they tend to run their fingers through their guy's hair. But the scalp is sensitive all the time, not just when you happen to be close to it. In some of the positions described later in the book, you'll be close enough to your man's head to lightly stroke his hair and scalp while fellating him. Some men also like to have their hair pulled (not hard enough to pull it out, but enough to create tension in the follicle) during orgasm. Is your man one of these? He may not know himself, so experiment with a few light tugs.

Armpits

Yes, they're stinky. But if you're willing to embrace the scent of manliness, armpits are jam-packed with nerve endings and tremendously responsive to stimulation. The very spot where you instinctively grabbed to tickle as a kid is the same place where thousands of nerve endings continue to hide out as an adult. The skin surrounding the armpits is delectably light and soft—explore it with your hands, fingers, tongue, and whatever else you can think of. Feather dusters (clean ones!), an individual feather, or an ice cube will work particularly well here. During oral sex, a couple of fingernails run from just below the belly button to the soft side of the upper torso and back again creates a cascade of sensations that will send some chills down his spine. It's nice to follow this move with a little nibble to the same area.

Below the Belly Button

Tickle and stroke this spot—perhaps continuing all the way down to the base of his penis—just as he's about to orgasm. Nine out of ten men will love it. One out of ten will be so busy climaxing that they won't seem to notice, but the added sensation will heighten their experience nonetheless.

The Sacred Sacrum

The sacrum is the large heavy bone at the base of the spine, roughly triangular in shape. I could write an ode entirely dedicated to this one little spot. But instead, I'll just tell you this: light, circular motions just before orgasm are divine here. Also, in the postcoital phase, stimulation on this little patch of sensitive, flat skin can lull your man into something of a trance. Just make sure to ask him questions to which you want the answer to be yes.

Fingers and Toes

Some people go wild for having their fingers or toes sucked, and it makes a great prelude to oral sex. Just remember that the skin between the fingers or toes is the most sensitive, and also be sure to play with the tips. For an extra erotic touch, hold your face right up to your partner's and make eye contact while you take their fingers into your warm, wet mouth. They'll figure out what's in store pretty quickly.

12

Understanding Your Man:
Using His Fantasies to Your Advantage

WHEN MAKING LOVE to a man, it can be important to keep some of the fundamental attributes of masculine psychology in mind. According to the stereotype, women are more likely to get turned off by an emotional failing than a slight physical flaw, while men tend to narrow their focus to the physical in sex without reacting as strongly to the emotional framework in which the sex is taking place. In other words, after a long and tedious argument, men will most likely still want to screw.

Though simplistic, the psychosexual hard-wiring does appear to fall roughly along such lines. Admitting that men approach sex—and oral sex—in a way that is different from the way women do can help you discover and engage your man's deepest and most powerful desires.

For starters, men get turned on when you compliment them on the body parts that they think are the most important. In a poll taken for a New York newspaper, one hundred men were asked which body parts they thought women found the most attractive. Their top three? Muscular chest and shoulders, muscular arms, and a big penis.

When the same amount of women were polled and asked what body parts they found most attractive on a man, they rated small and sexy buttocks first, slimness second, and a flat stomach third. The least valued characteristics for women were a big penis (these can be too big for some women), muscular chest and shoulders, and muscular arms!

Clearly, men and women think differently about what makes a man attractive. If you can figure out the body parts that he takes the most pride in and make sure to openly admire and caress them when he's undressing, in the shower, or as you slide off his clothes, the compliment will race to both of his heads.

In most surveys on the topic, the number of men who fantasize about sex "in a romantic setting" hovers around a meager 4 percent, and a whopping zero percent report fantasizing about "passionately kissing their partners." By contrast, fantasies about "being promiscuous" and "seducing an innocent" are reported to be around eight times more frequent in men than women. Of course statistics can't explain the nuances of individual behaviors, but here they do function to point out a general truth: woman and men tend to fantasize differently.

Men tend to fantasize about a particular group of situations and roles, all of which can be used in oral sex to heighten stimulation. These fantasies tend to engage issues of power, control, and ego—all aspects of character that are classically praised in men. Initiating sex without saying a single word, openly telling your partner how irresistible he is, playing dominant or submissive, or inviting a third party to participate is sure to tap into one of the central categories of your man's sexual psyche. Swearing unyielding, undying, profound, and faithful love—which may be the cherry on a woman's triple-scoop fantasy—does not appear nearly as frequently in men's sexual fantasies. In fact, in many situations such declarations during sex can easily lead to a sudden rush of blood from the small head to the big one.

Use your man's active sexual fantasizing to your advantage. Surprise him in a restaurant by squeezing his thigh and inviting him to the bathroom. Then give him a treat that will leave him dizzy through dessert. Whether you open the door to greet him as a French maid who speaks very little English, but who certainly knows how to make her agenda clear, or simply grab his crotch with a feistiness that's a little out of the ordinary, there's no way to underestimate the power of these heightening devices.

ROLE-PLAYING WITH ORAL SEX

Role-playing can provide an opportunity to be more playful and open to experimentation. Allowing you to step outside of your shyness and routine, role-playing can release you from your hesitations. Maybe you've never been brave enough to try deep throating, but Nancy the Naughty Maid does it without a care in the world. The most important aspect of this heightened sexual exchange is to be perfectly at ease with your partner and to have an open, communicative relationship—which means never doing anything against your will.

Role-playing is a way for the sides of us that aren't allowed expression in the day-to-day are given room to play. This makes it a great way to rejuvenate your sex life, because it opens the door to sides of your partner that you may not have known exist. The fact that your partner may have some pretty strange fantasies doesn't mean that he's sick, perverted, or twisted. Some surprising words

and impulses will probably come your way as well. Everyone has se-
cret fantasies and desires, and tapping into these can spark the dawn
of a new era in your sex life, or it can simply be a fun way to spend
the afternoon.

You can be:

The dumb blonde who just wants to screw.
The older-woman seductress luring him in.
The exhibitionist who lets him look up her skirt and fondle her in
public.
The boss who demands sex from her employee.
The maid who shows up for more than dusting.
An exotic nurse/bath attendant who learned some special tricks
chez elle.

The Striptease

For a gentle foray into this genre of sex play, you can treat him to a
striptease. Remember that a fully clothed woman and a fully nude
one are both a little less attractive than a scantily clad one. Music is
a must if this is your first time, because it will allow you to move
more rhythmically and detract from any feelings of awkwardness you
might have. After all, everyone dances in their underwear. Just make
sure to make plenty of eye contact and move your hips.

13

The Basic (Mind-Bending) Blow Job:
A Blow-by-Blow Account

THERE ARE ALMOST as many ways to initiate a BJ as there are men who love them. Here are a few suggested approaches, but remember that you know your man best, so feel free to mix and match.

When you're getting started, be practical: go ahead and take off your rings (especially if they have pointy jewels) and tie your hair back if it's long. Grab a cup of water, if there's one available, or some lubricant. Also, no matter where you are, make sure you seek whatever level of privacy makes you feel relaxed and sexy.

GENTLEMEN, START YOUR ENGINES . . .

The Silent, Sexy Approach

Don't say anything and simply go to your man with a knowing look in your eye. Begin kissing him, murmur how unbelievably sexy he is, and make sure to rub your breasts well into his chest and touch him intimately with your hands as you start to caress his hair, neck, and then his penis through whatever clothes he's about to take off.

Move decisively. Oral sex requires the performer to take charge, and a great way to start is by getting your man relaxed in the position that will be most comfortable for you. Once you start directing his motion to a nearby chair or bed, he's unlikely to put up much resistance.

The Teasing Approach

All too often, oral sex is initiated by sucking directly on the penis, as if there was only one goodie in the man store. However, with the single exception of the sudden quickie (where his orgasm is strengthened by delighted surprise), stronger, deeper orgasms are created by beginning with a tease. Or two.

Start by planting gentle, light kisses and nibbles on his inner thighs. A great deal of teasing can occur prior to this point, but the way you tease is more a matter of creativity than skill, so this aspect is up to you. By hook or by crook, once you've reached the genital area, it's time to start employing the more subtle arts of your tongue. The trick here is to move deliberately and slowly, even though you're coming on to him full speed and making him crazy with excitement. Give lingering kisses, and nibble your way down from the chest. Go about two steps slower than you know he wants you to.

Slowly enough to create some exquisite exasperation, but quickly enough to keep him aroused, allow your tongue to come at least two-thirds out of your mouth for a full lollipop-style lick around the perimeter of the genitals. This should be taken at a count of about one second per inch, and should not involve motion in your jaw. After this approach, retreat back down his thighs, leaving him twitching with desire.

THE GENITAL MASSAGE

A nice way to get a firm erection in place is by massaging his genitals—a delightful series of sensations that will get him hard if he isn't splitting his pants open already. Remember that males hit their sexual peak around age twenty (while women reach it closer to thirty—a cruel joke), so if your partner is significantly beyond his twenties you might need to cheer this one "up," so to speak, before hitting him with the magnum blasts you'll be learning later in the chapter.

To perform a great genital massage, start by rubbing and pressing his genitals from the outside of his pants with your hands or thigh. When you start to feel a response, slip down between his legs and unzip his pants. Reach in and touch him. If he's rock solid, he's dying for it and you can plunge right in. If he's soft, he might be a little nervous. Take his penis gingerly into one hand, and while pulsing it slightly between your palm and fingers, lean up and kiss him. A long, tongueful, sexy kiss. Is there any response from down below? Is there a little jolt through your hand? At this point, any movement is good movement.

SETTING HIS STAGE

Pull out his penis and grasp it firmly with one hand at the base (though not too firmly—hold the penis about as hard as you would a baby chick that you don't want to crush, but can't let escape from your hand). If it is entirely soft, use your hand to gently massage it upward, as if you are gently molding it into the desired erect shape. Remember that this is not necessarily a comment on his level of attraction to you. His desire may be off the charts; his penis isn't always going to comply. Don't act surprised. In fact, don't *be* surprised. Some guys just take a little longer to warm up.

Once he's semierect, hold his balls in one hand and his penis in the other. Squeeze him gently toward the bottom of the shaft while you coat your lips with plenty of saliva. Run your tongue all over your lips, until they're almost as wet as the inside of your mouth. Look up at him and make eye contact. Men are visual creatures, and who can blame them for wanting to watch such an intimate kind of pleasure?

FIND HIS HOT SPOTS

Learn from an Expert
To find out what he likes best, one direction you can take things in includes a little participation on his part. Squeeze some lube onto your hands and rub about half of it on his hands. This is a nice moment for hand play, and will warm the lube before you place your hands around his penis.

Place your hands in a praying position around his penis, making sure that your fingers are pointing at his chin and the tips are touching while your thumbs come upright together. You have to be between his legs for this one, as the exact angle of your hands is important. Once your hands are well positioned, ask him to place his hands around yours and control the motion and speed of your palms. Even if you speak different languages, this is sure to communicate exactly which types of touches—including pressure, speed, and direction—he likes most.

Search for the Holy Nerve Centers

Another option to find his hot spots is to simply go scouting for them yourself. The Lip Massage (page 38) has perfectly prepared you to locate the most jam-packed nerve centers on your man's pleasure wand. Every penis has its sweet spots—e.g., the glans or frenulum—but the exact location of the truly astounding sensation makers varies on every penis.

If your lips are both as soft and as they should be after performing the Jug of Plenty exercise (page 39), and as controlled as they should be after performing Button Up! (page 39), you should have no trouble conducting your hot-spot search. Avoiding the head for now, use light suction to pull about one-half inch of the skin of his shaft into the moist insides of your lips, and simply run along the edges of the shaft a few times. Some men have unusually sensitive spots here in places you wouldn't necessarily expect. Then move your light, mobile suction all around the base of the penis and the underside of the corona. Meanwhile, use your hands to provide rhythmic up-and-down motions. Scan the entire surface area of his penis for the spots that elicit the loudest sounds from him. Think of yourself as a metal detector—except you're looking for something more precious than pennies!

Once you've found a couple of spots that make him moan, twist a little, or knot up his eyebrows like he just had a difficult realization, he's putty in your hands. From here, you have a few choices on how to proceed.

THE LITTLE TEASE

When you're ready to begin taking him into your mouth, move your hands down to his balls and part your lips very, very slightly. Come very near his cock—but don't touch it yet! Look him in the eye as you get closer and closer. Continuously massage his balls with your hands, and don't stop until you absolutely need those hands for something else. Blow some hot, soft breath on him. Stick just the blade (the first third of your tongue) out and get even closer to taking him into your mouth. Once you're sure your tongue is dripping wet, start a long, soft stroke from the bottom of the shaft to the glans. Start on the underside, because this area is much more sensitive than the top.

On your way, it can be a fun addition to turn your head sideways and *pretend* to take a bite of him, *very gently* setting your teeth to touch his flesh.

When you reach the meatus, wet him again with your tongue, and use your lips to spread the moisture around if necessary. A wet cock sounds and feels much more erotic than a dry one, so don't skimp on the moisture.

Repeat several times, traveling up and down. Try to touch a different band of the shaft with every lick as you spread the sensations of warmth and moisture.

BACKSTAGE

Meanwhile, you may want to change your ball massage by lightly scratching them with the tips of your nails, changing direction or stroke style (from back and forth to a soft circular or sideways motion). You many also want to reach back behind his balls to get at that supersensitive area, the perineum. The muscle that causes erections originates here, so don't be surprised when this stimulation creates a major response in his penis.

KNOWING WHEN IT'S TIME TO MOVE ON

After you've licked his shaft enough times to make it sopping wet and acceptably hard, your man's going to start squirming if you don't get serious. Teasing is great, but keep checking his face to see when it's about to become too much. When he looks like he's squirming in line for the bathroom, things have gone too far. The first head toss or torso twist is the sign that it's time to get down to business.

THE RING

Now that you've licked him from bottom to top, on one of your upward strokes place the fingers of your right hand (or your left hand, if you're left-handed) in a ring formation at the base of his shaft. (If he's really big, it's okay to use both hands or a "double ring," but one hand is preferable because it allows you to keep engaging his balls and perineum.) Make the ring tight enough to completely conform to his shape, but loose enough to easily slide up and down. You want to keep this ring throughout your blow job, because it will stabilize the penis and give it the feeling of being completely encased when you take it into your mouth. When the ring is in place, use it to move up and down in time with your other motions.

GETTING DOWN TO BUSINESS

As you complete your upward tongue moves, keep going up and continue your warm, wet lick over the top of his cock. Linger at the meatus. With a sharp, pointed tongue, apply pressure to the meatus and try to stick your tongue into it if possible, while beginning to work your hand(s) up and down his shaft. But don't suck the head just yet. Run your tongue around the bottom of the corona, making frequent passes at the frenulum (this is the tender skin directly facing you).

THE COTTON CANDY STRETCH

Squeeze the shaft and look to see if any clear liquid comes out of the meatus. If some does, dip your tongue into it and then pull your head back. This precum will stretch with you and look incredibly erotic to your partner. Now that you have a long line of the stuff, dive back in like it's your favorite food and close in on the glans as if it were the head of an ice cream cone that you want to utterly devour. Take the entire head into your hot mouth, hold it between your lips for a few seconds, and listen to him moan.

THE GRAND ENTRÉE

This is getting to the part of the blow job that always gets close-ups in porno films, and for a good reason: it feels fabulous. With your tongue angled on the frenulum, take as much of his cock into your mouth as you possibly can, with your hand(s) firmly encircled around his base to compensate for whatever doesn't fit. If you bend your neck so that there is a straight line from his cock down your throat, you should be able to take in more than you thought.

Hold him deep within your mouth for a moment, and simply feel his strong cock inside your mouth, knowing that you are in no danger of losing your breath. If you learn to feel comfortable with it, this sensation can become fantastically erotic, and may eventually excite you as much as intercourse.

At this point, you can slide your lips to encircle the glans and flick your tongue against the frenulum. Your man will be getting restless, wanting more complete penetration, but don't let him run the show. He may think he wants it all right now, but then it would last only a few minutes and his orgasm would be below a five on a scale of one to ten. If you hold him at bay through a few more key moves, that baby will reach a ten out of ten every time.

HOW TO BUY YOURSELF SOME TIME

If your partner is already telling you (verbally or otherwise) that he feels the urge to ejaculate, grasp his penis and press your thumbs against it just beneath the glans. Maintain firm pressure for a few seconds. If this feels too clinical, you can cover your teeth with your lips, and use them to create the same effect.

WHISTLE WHILE YOU WORK

After you have taken him fully into your mouth and have started moving up and down the length of his shaft, make sure you use your tongue to lick all over the glans and frenulum while you're moving. Use the malleability of his cock against your warm, pointed tongue to experiment with certain focus areas (ideally the frenulum and corona) while you suck. You can rest the head of the penis on the roof of your mouth or in your cheek while you use your tongue to create more intense, precise sensations amid the general ones created by rhythmic sucking.

Those Pushy Hands

Your man may, at some point, press his hands on your head in an attempt to drive himself more fully into your mouth. This is an instinctual response—it's the same impulse that drives him to penetrate you more deeply at the moment of orgasm. Don't be offended by this gesture, but if it makes you uncomfortable, simply use your hands to gently nudge his away.

TAKE HIM TO THE EDGE...

Moving as fast as he can handle it, take him fully into your mouth (with the blade of your tongue pressed fully forward to maximize frenulum contact) and slide up and down his cock as rapidly as you can—*without* having him orgasm. If he comes close, slow down or even stop for a moment. Then, get back to it. Again, if you can't fit all of him in your mouth, use your hands to complete the sensation of deeper penetration. Just remember to keep your hands in time with your mouth.

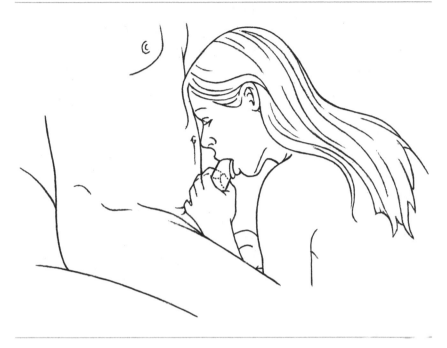

Ring Position

...AND PUSH HIM OVER IT

When he gets close to ejaculating, keep doing whatever got him to that point. Most men have orgasms from the rhythm of sucking on the head combined with the rhythm of the hand on the shaft and base of the penis. However, all men are different, and if another move has brought him to the cusp of climax, you can use that move just as easily to bring things to a head. If you have trouble identifying when he's going to climax, watch for the thrusting of the hips, moaning, the swelling of the glans, the clenching of the fists, and right before the climax you'll be able to feel what's coming in your right hand. For most men, a drop or two of fluid of extra precum will appear in the meatus immediately prior to takeoff. Of course, vocalizations ("Oh god, I'm gonna come") and mattress-slapping are pretty clear indicators.

Good Things Come to Those Who Wait

To get him to climax with more intensity, maintain positioning and light suction, while you *mange* him with nuzzling and massaging motions similar to those in the Button Up! exercise. Releasing the tension in your hands, but maintaining a firm lick, open your mouth to come up and over the head and take the entire penis into your mouth, including the shaft just beneath the corona.

Once here, your lips should first become light and airy, the closest thing you'll get to a literal "blow" job. This will send him into writhing bliss, especially if you lube up your lips, roll them out like in Pucker Up (page 35) and then pull upward so that your full, moist lips make contact with the entire underside of his corona. To drive him fully insane, press the blade of your tongue forward so that it makes extra contact with the frenulum.

Once you've done this a few times, surprise him with a pointed, aggressive tongue that dashes into his hot spot the moment you land on it, surrounded by the hot, juicy pressure of your lips, which are still conforming to his shape. Suck here about as hard as you would to keep a silver dollar stuck to your mouth, and top it off with a little pulling up over the glans. If he's uncircumcised, sandwich the glans in the shaft skin and take a few short up-and-down motions over the head to finish. Repeat a few times, and you've got a climax on your hands.

THE MOMENT OF TRUTH

When he's about to ejaculate, you have several options. Some people like to watch their men climax, because the visuals of spurting cum can be very erotic and exciting. If you want to watch, back off when you feel rising pressure in your right hand, and bring your (warm, lubed) left hand in to cover the head and participate in the rhythmic stroking. Squeeze pretty tightly with your left hand, and make sure your fingers and palm are positioned to give maximum sensation to the glans, perhaps closing the palm around the head of the penis on the upstroke, and allowing the head to break through the cushion between your thumb and forefinger on the downstroke. When he comes, turn your left hand into a ring, keep making contact with the corona and frenulum, and make sure the way is clear. For a parlor trick, you can try to catch some in your mouth if you're fast.

Another option that creates an erotic visual is to allow the warm, wonderful juices to gush up into your mouth, and then let them flow back onto his cock and slide around a little in the delightful mess. Running your hands up his wet shaft and over his glistening head is an intimate, sensual experience to be enjoyed by both of you. However, do this only once or twice since his penis may soon become painfully sensitive to the touch.

The Body Shot

Perhaps due to the proliferation of this image in porn, many men love to watch themselves come on their partners. If the taste displeases you, body shots can be an equally exciting prospect for him. Particularly good landing spots include the breasts, ass, or face (if at all possible—but if getting jizzed in the face isn't your idea of fun, the others are fine alternatives). Semen also tightens pores, so you'll get something out of it, too. A few encouraging words (e.g., "I love it when you shoot your hot, sticky cum all over me") can make this noningesting option even more exciting than the traditional swallow.

A Note on Swallowing

To swallow or not to swallow . . . that is the question. The sad truth is that cum can taste like anything from salty egg white to fish-flavored yogurt, neither of which appears on menus for a reason. If you simply can't stand the taste, take measures beforehand to circumvent the issue. You don't have to swallow, but you do have to be polite. Don't make your man feel like he has created something nasty or distasteful by getting up and running full speed to a sink, or by scrunching up your face like you just bit a rotting lemon. Keeping a couple of tissues handy to spit into should do the trick.

Men tend to identify themselves with their cum (it does, after all, contain their future generations) and this psychological association runs deep. Some men feel patently rejected when they see their partner spitting it out, while others don't particularly care. If you feel comfortable swallowing, it will most likely add to his pleasure. Simply taking the ejaculate into your mouth will set off some fireworks for him, because his receptivity to penile stimulation will peak in the nanoseconds preceding climax—an ideal time for you to be laying on your loving lips.

If you don't like the taste of semen, but want to take full advantage of the swallowing benefits, some of the deep-throat techniques discussed in the next chapter (see page 131) will be helpful to you. In deep-throat positions, the meatus (opening of the penis) is positioned beyond your taste buds, so that his cum will shoot straight into your throat. If that sounds a little intense for now, just make sure you're as cum-friendly as possible for as long as he's looking. Also, if you remove your lips and mouth just before he orgasms, be sure to immediately compensate with your hands and fingers.

If it's just the taste that bothers you, a modified technique is to insert the penis only slightly into your mouth and start swallowing immediately—and hard—right as he's beginning to come. If you can get it to the back of your mouth without inciting a gag reflex, you won't taste it at all. The fast-swallowing technique will also provide a delightful sensation for him at the height of his orgasm.

If you are comfortable with the idea of swallowing, know that studies have shown that, nutritionally speaking, semen is good for you, containing a cornucopia of vitamins and minerals, including vitamin B_{12}, calcium, magnesium, potassium, and even zinc.* You could be eating this stuff for breakfast.

If you don't know your partner well (or know that he is HIV positive), be sure to use protection and avoid swallowing, as taking his semen into your mouth puts you at risk of catching a wide variety of STDs.

All of the blow job techniques in this chapter will feel fantastic the first couple times, but it only takes a few repetitions for the penis to become desensitized to a particular stimulation. When you sense that this is starting, change your routine. You want his cock to be constantly on the brink of climaxing. Once you've got a raging hard-on in your right hand, and some tight balls in your left, it takes some new moves to stop those beauties from going to sleep.

---

* "Nutritional Value in a Serving of Semen." 2004 Columbia University's Health Q & A Service, © 2004 by the Trustees of Columbia University (http://www.goaskalice.columbia.edu).

14

Advanced Techniques

NOW THAT YOU have a road map of the most essential steps, find that one technique that can and will set him on fire.

SENSATIONAL SUCKING

There are almost as many different ways to suck as there are things to suck on. I've lost count of how many kinds I've come across, but here are a few to help you develop a repertoire.

The Cumming Circle
Place his hard cock in your mouth like you're going to start sucking—but don't tighten your lips around the shaft. Instead, making sure your lips are extremely moist, begin a circular motion with your head. Your teeth should be covered by your warm, wet lips. Switch between clockwise and counterclockwise motions, moving in a slow and stealthy manner. Make sure the bottom of your lips (rolled under to protect him from your teeth) makes contact with the coronal

ridge. If performed correctly, this technique can elicit multiple orgasms in men who are used to one-stop shopping.

The Pole Dance

Once you've found his sensitive spots, you can drive him further into a preorgasmic state that will lead to a more powerful orgasm without immediately provoking one.

To do the Pole Dance, position the taste bud side of your tongue a couple of inches below his hot spot, widen it, and fully apply it to the erect shaft so that the curve of your tongue completely adheres

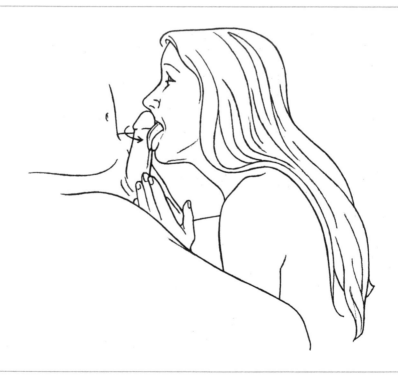

Pole Dance

to his curvature. Slowly move your tongue upward but not directly touching the spot you found. (If his hot spot is at the base, proceed directly to Pulling the Trigger, described in the next section.) Then, unless this gets a wild response that you want to explore, begin to twist and turn your deliberate, lickful self around and around his shaft, as if you're a tightly wound ribbon unwinding on his pole. The movements are long and circular.

This slow Pole Dance is an excellent time to lightly tickle and bandy your fingertips about on the undersides of his testes, his perineum, or his anus (if he likes that). In general, you want to contrast the sensations one part of you is creating (the intense, wide pressure of your tongue, in this case) with what the rest of you is doing (the light, playful dance of your fingers on his nether regions). Pole dance up and down, with varying speed, about three times. Pass over the hot spot as if you could care less. This is a great way to tease your man into a hungry, deeply aroused state.

Pulling the Trigger

If you've found some hot spots, but want to take him further into the outer realms of exhilaration before he climaxes, stave off the temptation to suck like mad. Instead, pull your mouth slightly back while using your hands to keep him stimulated (one firmly placed at the base of his penis, the other providing light up-and-down caresses). As you pull your mouth back, extend only the very tip of your pointed tongue to lightly explore the little gold mine you may have found. Use your pointed tongue to explore the area immediately surrounding it, and experiment with different pressure and strokes (pointed to wide) levels until you've found the spot where his body jerks like he's having a slight electric shock.

Now use just the most pointed tip of your tongue to give unbearably light, swift flicks to this specific area, while massaging his testicles.

The Butterfly Flutter

This famous move from porno films can easily be worked into your repertoire. The best position is for you to kneel between his legs. Or use the Going to Church position (page 150) and kneel in front of him while he stands.

This is a really sexy technique, because the positioning makes his cock feel thicker in your mouth, and you have more room to experiment with other areas with your hands. Essentially you are creating vacuum pressure on the cock with your mouth, but only enough to pull it slightly into your mouth.

Wrap your lips firmly around his hard cock. Make sure to cover the head and a little bit of the shaft. Gently flick the meatus (or just the tip in general will do) with your tongue. With your lips open just so that you can touch the tip of his cock with the tip of your tongue, make an up-and-down movement with your tongue without ever losing contact with the head. Essentially, you are fluttering your tongue in your open mouth over and over the frenulum. After several minutes, you can switch to a more basic blow job to finish him off.

Fun for Two

This is a variation for when you're ready to have some fun yourself. Go as far down on his cock as you can comfortably, with your lips firmly wrapped around his cock the entire time. Once you're down, open your mouth as wide as you can and suck in as much air as your lungs will let you. While sucking in this air, let your mouth travel up to the glans. The upstroke should end at his head just as your lungs are filling with air. With your mouth still open, let the air out of your lungs slowly through your mouth as you travel slowly back down the shaft.

This technique is fun and lighthearted, and incorporates temperature as his cock is cooled on the upstroke and warmed by your hot breath on the downstroke.

The Thirty-Second Orgasm

Of course it's not ideal, but sometimes you have to get your sweetie off in a hurry. This very easy way to do so simply requires a solid understanding of your partner's anatomy. Place your lips around the head of your partner's cock just beneath the coronal ridge, and wetly twist your lips around the corona alone at the back of the head of his penis. By sucking on this area of the cock continuously, you will produce a fast, forceful orgasm that doesn't even require you to bob up and down. The other great use of this technique is as a revitalizer when your man is flaccid but you want to play——a little bit of this stimulation will have him raring to go in no time.

Deep Throat

The average adult penis is five to six inches long when fully erect. The oral cavity of a woman is between three and four inches deep. Many of the techniques in this section have been passed down from the great fellatrixes of history (such as Cleopatra, who was particularly skilled in developing techniques to compensate for the difference). Unfortunately, more modern masters cannot be mentioned by name due to current libel laws.

In order to deep-throat correctly and comfortably, you need to study your own anatomy in addition to his. The primary obstacle is of course the ninety-degree angle behind your tongue that leads

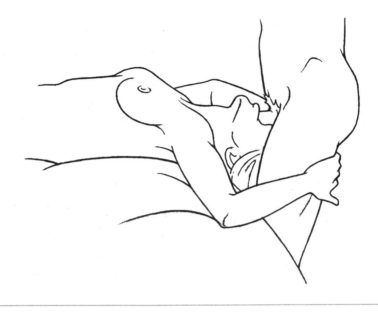

Deep Throating

down to your throat. The goal, then, is to get his penis past that an-gle, which is also past your gag reflex. If you don't want to swallow, make sure he's wearing a condom, because the positioning itself makes spitting out afterward a non-option.

Finding the Right Position
The most important aspect of any deep-throat position is that it al-lows for your throat and mouth to be in a straight line—this means leaning your head all the way back. Mastering the reaction to gag is the one and only trick to this position. Because of the way your mouth and throat are situated, he will be in control. You won't be

able to move or offer any stimulation other than that of keeping your mouth tightly closed around his fully inserted cock.

If you lie on a bed with your head on the edge, and tip your head sharply back, your lover will be able to insert more of his cock in your mouth—comfortably—than you ever thought possible. In fact, one of the greatest complications of this position is the tendency for pubic hairs to tickle your nose!

He needs to have his legs spread widely enough apart so that you have maximum movement and access. Maintaining this relaxation during the entire sex event is crucial, because in this position the man must generate *all* of the motion. He will move back and forth just like intercourse—except for the first time, he will be able to move as deeply into your mouth as he wants to. When you've mastered this position well enough to feel relaxed and comfortable, don't forget to use your hands to reach around and massage his buttocks and tickle his testicles.

If you have trouble mastering your gag reflex, work on completely relaxing your throat in the way described in the Tensing and Relaxing section of chapter 8 (page 74). You'll need to maintain this relaxation during the entire event, so make sure that you try this with someone you really trust, and approach it with a "practice makes perfect" attitude. Have him insert his cock inch by inch, while you relax your throat muscles, breathe through your nose, and find the most comfortable way to proceed. It is easiest to relax the throat muscles on the exhale of a deep breath. There is no room at all for him to move side to side, so when he's starting to climax you may want to place your hands on his hips to steady his motion.

Remember that it can take some couples the better part of a year to truly master this technique, so don't be discouraged if it takes some practice. Whether it is easy or hard for you and your partner has more to do with the shape of your anatomies than your skill as an oral lover.

Ice-skater

Once you've become comfortable with his cock very deep inside your throat, use this technique to cool your partner down a little without putting him to sleep. Quite the contrary, you'll be scraping him off the ceiling when you're through.

With your lips wrapped firmly around the shaft, try to reach the base. Go as slowly and steadily as you need to, using the principles of deep throating to guide you. When your nose is buried in, or at least touching, his public hairs, use your nose to trace three to four-inch figure eights on his cock. Let your nose lead your mouth and lips, which will stimulate his cock in just the right way. Keep doing figure eights all the way up and down his shaft. Your man is now realizing that the ultimate blow job is not only real—he knows where to get one.

When you get tired of this movement, slow it down and return to a basic move.

RIMMING

Before you engage your partner in anilingus, or "rimming," make sure that he is fresh and clean, preferably just out of the shower. Place a dental dam, opened condom, or plastic wrap over the area, with at least a couple inches to spare on each side. At no time should your tongue come into contact with the anus itself.

Place your partner on his back with his legs in the air and knees close to his shoulders. This is the position for maximum access. Although you might be under the impression that it's necessary to actually penetrate his anus to successfully perform anilingus, that's far from the case. In fact, unless you hit his G-spot (a few inches in toward the balls), very little is contributed to anilingus by penetration, since most of the nerve ending are located in the sphincter itself. Licking around the area, therefore, is even preferable to simply inserting the tongue. Anilingus is a powerful stimulant, and if you combine it with a well-tuned hand job, your man will have a rapid and powerful climax that he won't be forgetting anytime soon.

ADVANCED TESTICLE SUCKING

If your sucking of his testicles is combined with manual stimulation of his glans and perhaps even his nipples (this is possible from the classic position), extremely delightful sensations can be created. The testicles are easily hurt and very sensitive, so handle with care.

Ball Bath

Begin by gently licking his balls with your tongue, and as your partner warms up and becomes more passionate, take his nipples between your fingers and give them a light squeeze. Depending on his response, you may want to squeeze a little harder. Be very gentle so that he trusts you with his Twin Cities. Make sure to lick the balls all over to get the little hairs to lie down. Otherwise, you may inadvertently cause him pain by pulling on them with the movement of your mouth.

Tea Bagging

Lick the balls first with a well-moistened tongue, to encourage all of the tiny hairs to lie flat. You will need to keep your mouth wide open for the entirety of this technique, so I hope you've practiced the Side to Side, Up and Down, and Open Wide exercises from chapter 7. Once you have taken one or both of the testicles into your wide-open mouth, close only your lips to create very gentle suction; focus especially on rotating your tongue in circular motions on the underside of the balls to stimulate the place where the bottom of the testicles join the perineum. You can use your hands to stimulate your partner's penis, especially the soft head, and watch out for the fireworks.

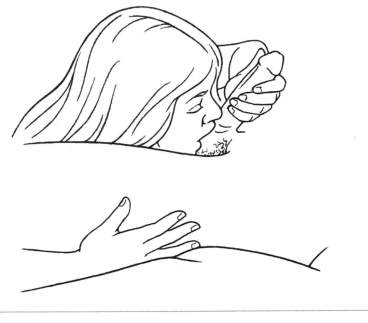

Tea Bagging

Lollipop Lick

Make sure your man is in an elevated position while you're on your knees facing him. Lift his cock to expose his balls. Using the tip of your tongue, find the underside of his balls where the skin joins the perineum. While resting his balls on your moist tongue, lick with an upward stroke to the tip of his cock. This technique is best performed in a succession of strokes, just like licking an oversized lollipop. Use flavored lube for a more complete rendition.

Few men can tolerate the lollipop lick for long without climaxing, so either limit this technique to three or four strokes, or save the lollipops for dessert.

HANDIWORK

Flexible and dexterous, the hands are an excellent sexual tool. Use a few of these techniques to put some variety in your handiwork.

Twist and (Listen to Him) Shout

You can keep one hand clasped firmly around the middle of the penis while cupping the other and rubbing your cupped palm over and around the head of the penis as if you were juicing a lemon. But instead of just twisting it from side to side, use your fingers and the angle of your hand to twist and pull upward at the same time, with your fingers stretching down for the beginning of the twist and gradually pulling up for a flourish at the end.

Break It Down

Place both your hands on the penis so that the majority of the shaft is covered. Now gently turn your hands in opposite directions around the shaft. Meanwhile, slip the index finger of your upper hand up onto the ridge of the glans; if your man isn't circumcised, pull a little foreskin up with you.

MISCHIEVOUS MISCELLANY

Here are a few extras that will drive him crazy regardless of what position you're in, what time of day it is, or where you are. These tips are made to travel.

The Kiss of Life

When he's in need of major revitalization, use the Kiss of Life. Once your man has ejaculated, you're going to have a hard (no pun intended) time getting him to ejaculate again. Use this technique to get him hard enough to climax again (and again and again).

Beyond the Thirty-Second Orgasm technique of stimulating the coronal ridge, you're going to need to do more than simply stimulate his genitals to elicit a second (and third, and fourth) orgasm. Although you can get him hard again, you still have a good stretch of road ahead of you before he can climax again. Combine some of the basic techniques to get the juices flowing, but the best idea for the second and third rounds is to explore the rest of his body.

This is a particularly delicious moment in oral sex—since there's no pressure to make him climax, you can take your sweet time touching every square inch of his body with your tongue just to see what effect it has. If you haven't been stimulating these much so far, use this time to pay some attention to his nipples and his earlobes, his perineum, balls, and anus, as well as the backs of his knees, toes, fingers, neck, navel, and sacrum. (Review chapter 11 for a more in-depth look at other erogenous zones.)

The second round is a perfect time to introduce a sex toy—from feather to ice cube to vibrator—to get him interested and ready for another go-round.

How to Put on a Condom with Your Mouth

While the condom is still in its wrapper, quickly make sure that it has an air bubble inside the wrapper (otherwise it might be punctured) and check the expiration date. If these make the cut, very gently

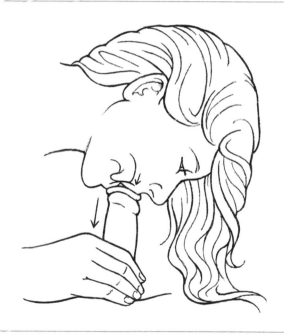

Putting a Condom on with Your Mouth

open the package, being especially careful not to press too hard if you have long nails. Pinch the condom by the tip (and make sure you're not holding it upside down, especially if you've had a few drinks). Place the entire condom in your mouth, with the ring behind your teeth and your tongue pressed against the reservoir tip.

The blade of your tongue should be flattened wide enough to cover the entire tip. With the condom in your mouth, drop a little lube on your guy's tip. If you're concerned about the taste, use one that's flavored. Lower your head, and use your tongue to press out all the air from the reservoir tip against his glans. This can be a fun opportunity for a little frenulum action as well. When your tongue has pressed out all the air, release the ring of the condom and place your lips above it, unrolling it down the length of his shaft on one long, gently pressing motion. Conform your lips to his shape, but be careful not to bite. Too hard.

Orgasm Catalyst

To take your blow jobs to the next level, place your thumb at the base of the penis so that the tube through which the semen ejaculates is blocked. If your thumb is placed correctly, the semen will not be able to release even though your man will be spasming and otherwise experiencing every aspect of a full-fledged climax.

While you're holding your thumb in this position, suck the glans with some serious verve. When you finally allow the semen to release, his ejaculation will last much longer and will be much more intense than any standard orgasm. Even if you delay it for just a few moments or seconds, you'll be surprised at the intensity of the resulting ejaculation. But not as surprised as he is!

THE JOYS OF TOYS

Some toys are definitely *not* made for children. Introducing these into the bedroom can add a whole new dimension to your sex life, and can make oral sex more exciting—and a whole lot more pleasurable.

Mini-Vibrator

Start with a vibrator about four inches long and three-quarters inch in diameter. To soften the sensations, consider buying a soft, penis-shaped plastic sleeve. While fellating your partner, use any of the oral techniques described earlier while enhancing the sensations with the added stimulation. As an extra sexy bit of foreplay, run the exposed plastic vibrator up and down the bottom of the penis, and make gentle circles around the frenulum, creating deeply satisfying stimulation. The vibrator can be used to touch, stroke, and tap anywhere on the perinium, testicles, anus, or on the shaft itself.

The most intense feelings of pleasure possible for a man can be created by performing fellatio while pressing a (well-lubricated) vibrator into your partner's anus very slowly and gently. It is very important to move slowly, since the inside of the anus is delicate domain. However, if you insert the vibrator fully, its tip will just barely touch the prostate (the man's G-spot), which is more than enough to revolutionize his oral sexual experience. Some men prefer an in-and-out motion with this technique, but others prefer the vibrator to lie still. Still others like a gentle pulsing motion somewhere between the two.

The best position for this technique is for him to be on the floor or bed with legs bent and knees high, while you are between his knees in whatever position gives you access to his entire range of

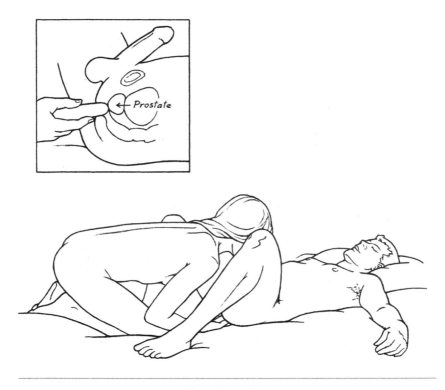

Three-Ring Circus

genitalia. For some, this will be with him lying on his back; for others, the best way is for him to lie on his side with your head resting between his legs.

Modified Doggie

Some men find it more comfortable to accept the vibrator from a doggie-style position, resting their arms and upper body on a bed-post or other support while you are in a sitting position below them. This is a great position in front of a mirror, because your man can get awesome views of your hardworking tongue and lips, which he is going to love.

A nice element to throw in here would be a light but rhythmical butt massage with your palms, and some gentle stroking of the testicles (if your partner finds this pleasurable—if he's the kind who wants his orgasm NOW!, lay off as usual). Make sure to use the hand you write with to manipulate the vibrator in this case, because control and access to the prostate are essential.

Tip: You may want to support your lower back with pillows, as few men tire of all the advantages to be gained by this position.

15

Oral Sex Positions:
The Hot and the Twisted

MEN ARE EROTIC visualists and primarily aroused by what they can see (one reason why they're so into porn). So when you're choosing a position, make sure to select one where they can see the action. No matter which position you're in, let him see your face or even hold your hair back. Keep your eyes open, and turn your man on by making eye contact occasionally as you're going up and down his shaft.

THE CLASSIC POSITION

An excellent starting position is for him to be seated in a comfortable chair or on a sofa with his legs spread wide, while you kneel (ideally on a pillow or rolled-up towel) in front of him. Make sure that his hips are far enough toward the edge of the chair so that you have a good range of access. The best positions will always be those in which you approach him from the bottom of his penis rather than lying alongside him or approaching him from the side or top, because the underside of his penis has the most nerve endings.

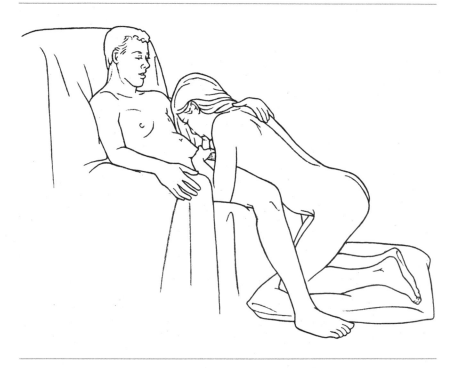

Classic Position

POWER POINT

If you find that your partner is most sensitive all the way around the corona (some are most sensitive only on the underside), a good position is for him to sit halfway up on the side of a bed with his legs hanging off the side. You can kneel on the floor alongside him so that your head is about level with his chest. This is essentially the Classic Position, but instead of coming at him from the front, you are approaching him from the side. The benefit is that, by using one arm around him to support yourself, you can achieve very rapid strokes in this position. Make sure, however, that your fingers maintain contact with the frenulum the entire time you're in this position (because you aren't approaching him from where the majority of his nerve endings are).

From this position, he can use a free hand to stroke your hair, pinch his (or your) nipples, and caress and stimulate his testicles and

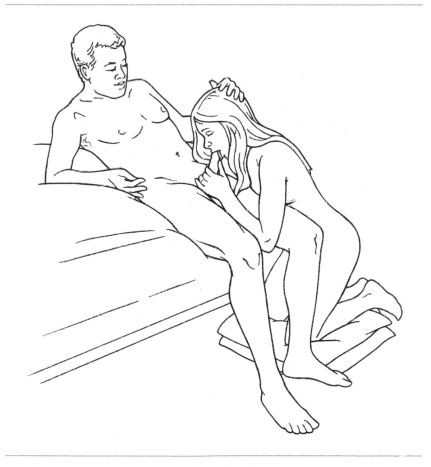

Power Point Position

shaft while you give him oral sex. This can be a great way to experiment with what he likes together, because when you approach from the side, you both have room to participate.

THE SWING OF THINGS

If you need to switch to a position that will relax the muscles of your neck and back, and happen to be on a large enough surface or can get to one, switch to the Swing of Things. In this position, he is lying back and just relaxing. You are in a modified 69 position over him, with your legs to one side. Wrap one arm under the thigh closest to you, so that you can provide stimulation to his perineum, his testicles, and the sensitive skin surrounding these areas. With the other hand, make sure that your index and middle finger make good contact with the other side of his penis, because the frenulum will still need to be stimulated.

This position is great for using the ridges along the top of your mouth to stimulate the juncture beneath the corona, where the various types of skin come together. Also, you can make the most of the soft, gentle contact between your chest and his abdomen, perhaps initiating a soft rocking or "swinging" motion that some men love. Make sure that your mouth is open wide enough to avoid any contact with your teeth, perhaps covering them with the skin of your lips to avoid chafing. This position requires a good bit of lubrication, but the benefits are worth it.

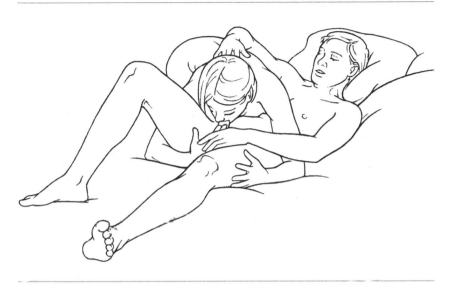

The Swing of Things

MAN'S ALL-TIME FAVORITE POSITION

If it came down to a matter of voting, this position would probably win. The man lies back and enters a fully receptive mode, without even flexing his knees. You bend over him—ideally from below—and give him oral sex from above. Though it does little for your comfort, the total comfort on his part does help him relax and focus on the pleasure you're giving him.

This position is best for a long, leisurely Sunday blow job. You can take your time, reach up and easily play with his nipples, caress his legs and thighs, and generally have enough freedom of movement so that the only limits are those of your imagination.

GOING TO CHURCH

In this position, the man is standing up and leaning against a wall and you are on your knees. Ideally, depending on your relative heights, your big head is just above his little one, so that by leaning slightly forward your lips will touch the tip of his penis and beyond (yes, you will look like you're praying, and yes, that is how this position got its name).

One of the several benefits of this position is the psychological impact on the man when he sees you in such a wholly compliant and giving position, 100 percent focused on his pleasure. While your feminist friends might puke at the notion, the likelihood is that it will turn him on in a major way. And if you don't get the gist of that, have him perform oral sex on you while kneeling in front of you, and see if your legs don't turn to Jell-O.

In this position, guys can get so excited and orgasmic that their legs will routinely begin to shake. Don't be scared—they rarely actually fall.

SWORD SWALLOWER

In this position, the man stands with one leg slightly forward and bent, while the woman is on all fours in front of him. As the name suggests, it's an excellent position for deep-throat techniques. Sword Swallower allows the woman both total access and more control than other deep-throat positions. The alignment of the neck to the penis allows the woman to easily take in a longer penis. A pillow under your hands and knees is a nice touch.

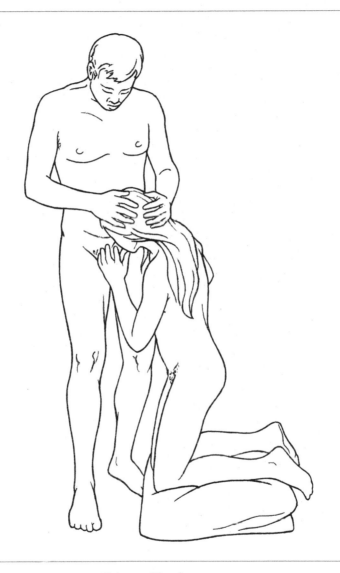

Going to Church

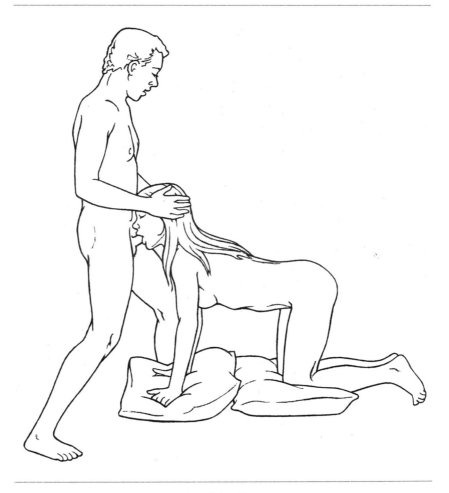

Sword Swallower

MUTUAL LOVE-FEST

In this pleasure-for-two scenario, the man kneels on the edge of a bed (or other raised surface) while you stand on the floor with one leg propped up on the side of the bed (usually on the bed frame).

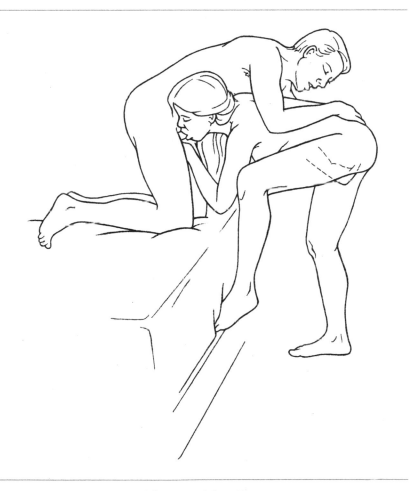

The Mutual Love-Fest

Once you're in position, give him oral sex focusing on the head. While your hands gently massage his balls, he will be more than happy to return the digital pleasure.

WINE ME, DINE ME, 69 ME

A nice variant of the 69 for oral sex is for both of you to lie on your sides, with your head down between your partner's legs. This is a terrific position for a partner who likes butt play, and while you stimulate his perineum and anus with your mouth (and a dental dam), you can squeeze your breasts together to give his penis the feeling of penetration.

Conclusion

HE BIGGEST SURPRISE to oral sex is how much you are going to enjoy taking your partner to these extremes of pleasure. The greater the arousal you produce in them, the greater the arousal you are likely to feel. When performed by someone skilled and confident in their abilities, oral sex is a concrete example of the pleasure of giving. The greater the degree of delight you produce within their body, the greater your own will be able to experience. Just witnessing the kinds of orgasms sparked and kindled by the exercises and techniques in this book is a fantastic experience. If you truly utilize what you have learned here, you may see men pulling their own (and your) hair, ripping pillows, sheets, their clothing (and your T-shirt if you're wearing one), screaming a wide variety of words (some expletives) and closing their eyes to lose themselves in the pleasures that will beckon them. Furthermore, after these orgasms the recipient tends to become quite giving in nature for at least several hours, and sometimes days. Do not abuse this indulgent attitude toward you, but feel free to enjoy it.

> Smile—it's the second best thing you can
> do with your lips.
> —ANONYMOUS

ABOUT THE AUTHORS

MARCY MICHAELS is a consulting speech pathologist/audiologist and educator with over twenty-five years' experience in her field. She has worked with a broad and diverse clientele, ranging from actors and broadcasters to international businessmen and children. She has four degrees in speech and biology, including a premed program at NYU, a BS in speech and communication arts from Adelphi University, an MS in speech pathology and audiology from Long Island University, and a postgraduate degree in speech education from St. John's University. She lives in New York City.

MARIE DESALLE attended the Sorbonne, then graduated from Sarah Lawrence College in New York with a BA in writing. Her interest in sex has manifested itself in photography, writing, and other artistic forms of self-expression. She lives in New York City.